Progress in Orthopaedic Surgery

Vol. 3

The Knee: Ligament and Articular Cartilage Injuries

Edited by D. E. Hastings

Contributors
W. Bandi, Interlaken · D. Baumann, Munich · C. Burri, Ulm
H. Cotta, Heidelberg · R. Ganz, Berne · W. Glinz, Zurich
L. Gotzen, Hannover · M. H. Hackenbroch, Munich
M. Häring, Freiburg · G. Helbing, Ulm
H. R. Henche, Rheinfelden/Baden · P. Hertel, Homburg/Saar
I. Hesse, Hannover · W. Hesse, Hannover · E. H. Kuner, Freiburg
L. Leichs, Munich · E. Morscher, Basel · J. Müller, Liestal
W. Müller, Basel · G. Muhr, Hannover · W. Puhl, Heidelberg
H. J. Refior, Munich · J. Rehn, Bochum · A. Rüter, Ulm
I. Schneider, Bochum · L. Schweiberer, Homburg/Saar
W. Spier, Ulm · D. Terbrüggen, Freiburg
H. Tscherne, Hannover · H. Willenegger, Berne

With 139 Figures

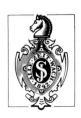

Springer-Verlag
Berlin Heidelberg New York 1978

Guest Editor: D. E. Hastings, Suite 613, 1849 Yonge Street, Toronto, Ontario M4S 1Y2, Canada

ISBN 3-540-08679-X Springer-Verlag Berlin Heidelberg New York
ISBN 0-387-08679-X Springer-Verlag New York Heidelberg Berlin

Library of Congress Cataloging in Publication Data. Reisensburger Workshop zur Klinischen Unfall-chirurgie, 3d–4th, 1975. The knee. (Progress in orthopaedic surgery; v. 3) Selected papers of the 3d and 4th Reisensburg Workshop held Feb. 27–Mar. 1, and Sept. 25–27, 1975. Includes biblio-graphies and index. 1. Knee – Wounds and injuries – Congresses. 2. Ligaments – Wounds and injuries – Congresses. 3. Articular cartlage – Wounds and injuries – Congresses. I. Hastings, David Erich, 1932– II. Bandi, W. III. Title. IV. Series.
RD561.R44 1975b 617'.14 78-5344

Typesetting, printing and binding: E. Kieser KG, Augsburg
2120/3321 543210

Contents

The Acute Cartilage Injury   95

The Old Cartilage Injury   121

Retropatellar Cartilage Degeneration   143

Preface

The editorial group has selected these papers for publication in *Progress in Orthopaedic Surgery* from contributions to the "Reisensburg Workshop of Clinical Trauma Surgery" dealing with the lesions of knee ligaments and cartilage in 1975. They represent a survey of today's knowledge of pathophysiology, diagnostic means, and therapy of these lesions in the German-speaking countries.

There are two "Reisensburg Workshops" annually, covering current topics of traumatology sponsored by the Ulm trauma group. Primary attention is focused not upon review lectures but rather upon the extensive discussions thus resulting in recommendations to the practising trauma surgeon in order to facilitate his clinical work.

Ulm, November 1977   C. Burri, A. Rüter

Introduction

This volume of *Progress in Orthopaedic Surgery* presents a selection of papers dealing with injuries to the ligament support and articular surfaces of the knee. The menisci are not discussed as separate entities, but rather in their correct perspective as part of the knee joint support mechanism. As the editor for this volume, I have tried to select the most representative articles which cover this subject. These are publications from our European colleagues and reflect their opinion and experience. I have tried not to change their content or meaning in any way. This volume has been divided into six basic segments. Each deserves comment.

The concept of the four-jointed chain system is a difficult one to grasp, but is sound on an engineering basis. It is clear from this key interaction of the cruciate ligaments how the loss of one cruciate will lead to a profound alteration in knee mechanics. Many authors suggest that the loss of stability from an isolated anterior cruciate ligament may be minimal, but I think that this article demonstrates the possibility of severe complications occurring in the later stages. Changes in articular cartilage detected under electron microscopy are irreversible after a short period of immobilization, especially in full extension. This experimental work reinforces the potential value of the cast brace or limited motion plaster.

The acute knee ligament injury is discussed only briefly in this volume. Unfortunately there was no article which adequately stressed the major problem with the acutely injured knee, namely the recognition of the severity of the original injury. The vast experience accumulated by North American surgeons on reconstructing chronically unstable knees suggests that our treatment of the acutely injured knee is less than optimal. The "relatively" isolated anterior cruciate tear that shows a history of a pop and a rapid hemarthrosis is seldom recognized. Severe disruptions including the medial ligament complex and the anterior cruciate ligament are often missed and lead to late complex instability. The treatment of the isolated collateral tear is still controversial. Even in Europe there is debate as to whether the optimal treatment is operative repair or immobilization. The diagnosis of such an injury often requires a general anesthetic to rule out an associated cruciate lesion. If the collateral lesion is isolated, then I would feel that many can be managed nonoperatively and that the limited motion plaster presents an ideal technique for this.

Chronic knee ligament instability is a subject that is familiar to most orthopaedic surgeons in North America. The concept of rotational instability has gained wide acceptance on both sides of the ocean. Many tissues are available for reconstructing the unstable knee. Certainly the pedicle graft using the biceps on the lateral side, a portion of the pes on the medial side, and portions of the patellar tendon for cruciate problems are all valuable adjuncts to a capsular repair. Of particular interest to me was the use of skin as an autologous ligament substitute. Although the authors have not carried out a large number of reconstructions over the years, their results appear acceptable. The use of skin could be an adjunct to other pedicle grafts in severe ligament disruptions. This is an area for further exploration and experimentation.

Acute injuries to the articular surface of the knee are often underestimated in comparison with meniscal or ligament damage. The series of papers dealing with this subject clearly show that the shearing injuries removing either a cartilage cap from the underlying subchondral bone or the more common osteochondral fracture can be replaced and will heal, restoring a normal cartilage surface. The entity of cartilaginous impression of the femoral condyles is an interesting concept. It is difficult to determine when it is a normal anatomic variant or a pathological entity.

Drs. Hesse and Hesse have presented very clearly an experimental basis for cartilage transplantation. In particular their meticulous work on electron microscopy suggests that the cell death in homographs is not visible by normal histologic methods. On the other hand, autologous cartilage transplantation from adjacent areas should stand a high chance of success. this is obviously why the replacement of an osteochondral fragment and large areas of osteochondrosis dissecans are likely to meet with success. The secure fixation of these fragments and the early motion of the knee are clearly the two main factors that ensure success.

The entity of chondromalacia and subsequent patellofemoral arthritis remains a common and difficult problem. The diagnosis is often not as easy as might be suggested. All the authors, however, stress the importance of two basic etiologic factors, an abnormal gliding pathway or an abnormal gliding surface. The toughness of articular cartilage appears to be due to the tangential fibers on its surface. Once these are unmasked by shaving, the concept of increased pressure accelerating wear must be considered. Anterior displacement of the tibial tubercle combined with retinacular release appears to offer the most efficient method of dealing with the problem.

This third volume of *Progress in Orthopaedic Surgery* has tried to follow the aims of previous issues. The work of our German-speaking colleagues should be shared with their North American counterparts, so that each may profit from the other.

Toronto, November 1977   D. E. Hastings

Biomechanics and Pathophysiology

The Biomechanics and Pathophysiology
of the Knee Ligaments

P. Hertel and L. Schweiberer

Biomechanics

Terminal Rotation (The Screw Home Mechanism)

From full flexion to full extension the femoral condyles and tibial plateaus move
in the sagittal plane during active motion. In the terminal stage of extension,
there is also a rotational movement in the horizontal plane. This [13] rotation
reaches about 10° in full extension. Firmly fixed on the ground, the foot
represents internal rotation of the femur on the tibia, when free it represents
external rotation of the tibia. When the active knee stabilizers are completely
relaxed, terminal rotation leads to maximum tightening of all passive stabilizers.
This rotation movement is partially controlled by the ligament system [5, 15]
and partially by the joint surfaces [16]. Although the joint surfaces and capsular
ligament systems function optimally together during terminal rotation, the dissected specimen shows that this phase can be maintained with light axial compression without any ligament support, even after division of the cruciate ligaments.

Terminal rotation corresponds to the direction in which the lower leg turns
spontaneously after division of the capsular ligaments. When divided, the cruciate ligaments unwind from each other, lie parallel, and their full length is exposed [6]. Loosening of the cruciate ligaments during terminal rotation is
necessary because of the noticeable rise of the anterior tibial plateau contact
surfaces on extension, especially on the medial side [13], and the anterior elon-
gation of the femoral radii of curvature.

Axis of Movement of the Knee Joint

Knee flexion in the sagittal plane does not represent a continuously centered
hinge motion as, e.g., the elbow joint. In fact, the various centers of curvature

of the femoral condyle can be easily determined. They proceed along a line that shows an increase in length of the radii of curvature in the direction of extension. The centers of the curvature of the femoral condyle, however, do not correspond to the axis of motion of the knee joint. The axis of motion can be easily traced if the knee joint is compared to a mechanical system, a so-called closed, planar, kinetic, four-jointed chain or four-bar linkage [9, 15, 20]. Such a classification carries two prerequisites:

1. The motion must be carried out in only one plane; this applies to the knee with the exception of terminal rotation.

2. The joints of the four-jointed chain must be rigidly connected. This applies to the system: cruciate ligaments, tibia, and femur inasmuch as in all positions some of the fibers in both cruciate ligaments are under tension.

Four-Jointed Chain System (Four-Bar Linkage)

The closed four-jointed chain has, as suggested, four joints connected by four rigid segments. By definition the planar, closed four-joint chain moves in one plane, and these movements can easily be demonstrated on drawing paper (Fig. 1).

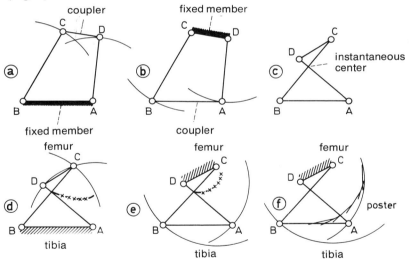

Fig. 1. (a) ABCD is a closed four-bar kinematic chain, which moves in the plane of the paper. If AB is the fixed member, all points on AD and BC move on circular arcs about A and B respectively. Points on CD, the coupler, (other than C and D) move on coupler curves which are not circular arcs (b) Each member of the four-bar chain can be the fixed member (c) This crossed, closed, four-bar chain corresponds to the anatomic structure of the cruciate ligaments (AB the intercondylar eminence of the tibia, BC the anterior cruciate ligament, AD the posterior cruciate ligament, DC the intercondylar fossa of the femur). The axis of motion of the knee passes through the instantaneous center, the crossing-point of the cruciate ligaments (d, e) Depending on whether the tibia or the femur is regarded as the fixed member, different loci of the instantaneous center result (f) When the tibia is moved relative to the fixed femur, the successive positions of the coupler yield a coupler envelope curve as shown

They are defined by a change of one segment, whereby one of them (the supporting link) maintains its position while the other three segments change position. The end point of the supporting link represents the centers of motion of all points of the adjoining members, while the points of the link opposite to the supporting link, the so-called coupler performs noncircular movements, the so-called coupler curves (Fig. 1a and b).

The cruciate ligament system, therefore, resembles a crossed, closed, planar four-jointed chain (Figs. 1c and 3). CD corresponds to the intercondylar fossa of the femur, AB to the tibial eminence, and BC and AD to the anterior and posterior cruciate ligaments respectively. The center of the axis of the knee joint conforms to the crossing point of link BC and AD and is called the "pole" or instantaneous center. During knee flexion the instantaneous center moves dorsally on its pole curve. Depending on whether the femur or tibia represents the supporting segment, two different pole curves can be traced with ruler and compass (Fig. 1d and e).

Design of the Femoral Condyle

Another curve can be derived from the motion of the four-jointed chain. Insertion of the anterior and posterior cruciate ligaments at the tibia represent approximately the altitude curve of the joint surface of the tibial condyles. With the femur fixed the tibial joint surface becomes the coupler. During knee flexion the locus of the midpoint of the coupler is a curve corresponding to the contour of the femoral condyles (Figs. 1f and 2a).

Points of Contact: Rolling and Gliding

All points of the coupler move with an instantaneous velocity directed perpendicularly to the radius from the instantaneous center. Since the velocity at the femorotibial contact point corresponds to the direction of the tibial joint surface, the point of contact must always lie perpendicularly below the instantaneous center, i.e., below the crossing of the cruciate ligaments. Therefore, by constructing a pole curve, it is possible to arrive at a geometric determination of the contact points between femur and tibia during various positions of flexion. This is done by drawing the normal from the pole to the coupler. By marking the contact points on the tibia in succession (Fig. 2) the combined gliding and rolling movements typical of the knee joint can be demonstrated. A purely rolling motion never occurs. In pure rolling, the distances between two points of contact on the tibia and femur would become equal. This occurs only during the primary phases of flexion; with increasing flexion the contact points at the tibia condyle are drawn increasingly together. If there were a purely gliding motion, only one point of contact would exist on the tibial segment.

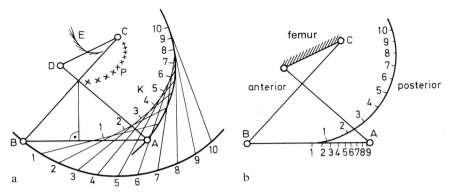

Fig. 2. (a) 10 different positions of the coupler AB were drawn between the circular arcs with radii BC and AD. The resulting coupler envelope curve K corresponds to the contour of the femoral condyle. The 10 corresponding instantaneous centers produce the pole curve P. The contact points of the coupler are determined by the normals through the appropriate instantaneous centers. The continuations of these normals yield the evolute E (locus of the center of curvature of the femoral condyle). (b) If the distance along the coupler to the contact point in each of the different positions of flexion is marked on AB, the corresponding points on the femur and tibia result. The fact that as flexion increases these points are more closely grouped posteriorly shows the predominance of sliding motion in squatting

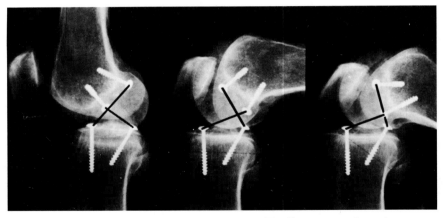

Fig. 3. The kinematics of the cruciate ligaments. The ligamentous insertions are marked by screw heads. In the extended positions the position of the four-jointed chain of Figs. 1 and 2 is visible. The angular motion of each cruciate ligament is considerably less than that of the femur

Anatomic – Functional Observations

The femorotibial connective soft tissue segments have to be considered passive stabilizers of the knee and are situated more posteriorly. The quadriceps, the main dynamic stabilizer, occupies the anterior surface (Fig. 4). Besides the well-described major ligaments of which the posterior cruciate stands out as the central stabilizer [1, 2, 7] the capsular ligaments have received more attention

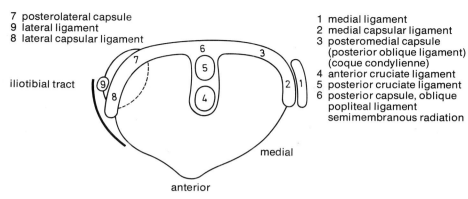

Fig. 4. Schematic drawing of the passive stabilizers in a top view of the right tibial joint surface. The passive stabilizers comprise the entire circumference of the posterior half of the knee. The capsular ligaments serve important stabilizing functions

recently. On the medial side, these include the deep layer of the medial ligament which holds the medial meniscus in place and stabilizes external rotation movements [17] and the posteromedial capsule, which primarily enhances medial stability while surrounding the medial femoral condyle and tibial plateaus like a ribbon [3, 8, 17]. The French literature terms this the "coque condylienne" and the American literature, the "posterior oblique ligament". It should not be confused with the oblique popliteal ligament, which represents a continuation of the semitendinosis muscle and serves to reinforce the strong posterior capsular ligament.

A similar posterolateral, ribbonlike portion of capsule is present between the femoral and tibial condyles. It is interrupted, however, by the popliteus tendon. The lateral capsular ligament can − like the medial − be divided into a menis-cal-femoral and meniscal-tibial segment. In addition there are superficial ramifications of the iliotibial tract laterally. Consequently passive stabilization is enhanced because of its connection with the distal femur via the lateral inter-muscular septum.

The entire passive stabilization system is tight during hyperextension. During flexion the lateral ligaments, the posterior capsule, and the posterior portion of the medial ligament lose their tension. The anterior portion of the medial ligament, however, remains tense during the range of flexion. Tension of the cruciate ligaments decreases in the early stages of flexion and increases again as the fibers twist during full flexion [1, 2].

Pathophysiology of Ligamentous Instability

Several methods have been used for pathophysiological examination of the knee ligaments.

1. Quantitative: Ligamentous tension can be measured directly by using a stretch measuring tape. Engin and Korde [4] reported lateral tension in varus

and valgus deformities of 2.5° and 5° under increasing axial loading. The tension of the medial ligament under additional pressure increased only in a valgus position of 5°. In other positions (valgus 2.5°, varus 2.5°, and 5°) only a slight change in the collateral ligament tension occurred under increased axial load.

2. Qualitative: This method can be demonstrated in artificially produced injuries. As early as 1877 Hönigschmied described the damaged anatomic structures after hyperextension, rotation, etc. He also made localized ligamentous lesions by specific sectioning and correlated this to the ensuing loss of stability [1, 3, 6, 11].

We prepared 16 fresh knee ligament specimens without prior injury. These specimens were mounted and the medial and lateral sides labeled separately. The individual passive stabilizers were dissected step by step and examined radiologically. Up to 40 radiographs were taken on each knee.

Isolated Ligamentous Instability

Isolated Lesions of the Cruciate Ligaments

The anterior and posterior cruciate ligaments can show signs of local instability [11, 14]. After experimental sectioning of the anterior cruciate ligament, the anterior drawer sign increased 2–6 mm. Sectioning of the posterior cruciate ligament resulted in a posterior drawer of 13–15 mm. The peripheral capsular ligaments resulted in restricting further motion (Fig. 5). Varus and valgus positions and hyperextension remained unchanged. Passive hyperextension occurred only after division of the posterior capsule, particularly the posterior part of the medial ligament. Isolated injury to the anterior cruciate ligament can occur without showing definite clinical symptoms.

Individual Lesions of the Collateral Ligaments

Individual lesions of the collateral ligaments occur in varus valgus or rotational injuries. The maximum load is exerted on the peripheral segments [10].

Valgus Instability

Injuries involving the whole medial capsular ligamentous apparatus result in a greater degree of medial instability than medial ligament injuries alone. A clean valgus injury can be imitated by step by step sectioning, starting with the medial ligament, the medial capsular ligament, the posteromedial capsular ligament, and finally the anterior cruciate ligament (Fig. 6). Such sectioning permits the objective demonstration of increasing instability and is the sequence followed by

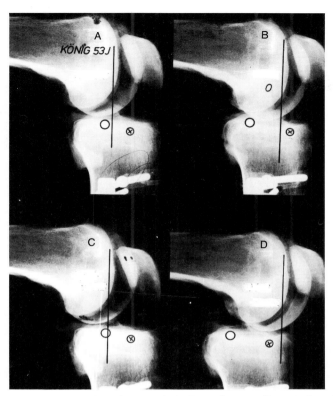

Fig. 5. *A* anterior drawer sign, knee intact; *B* posterior drawer sign, knee intact; *C* anterior drawer sign, anterior cruciate divided; *D* posterior drawer sign, posterior cruciate divided; ⊗ medial tibial plateau; ○ lateral tibial plateau. The range of motion of the lateral tibial plateau (measured against a line perpendicular to the anterior femoral cortex) is greater than the medial in the intact knee. Division of the anterior cruciate ligament allows an anterior tibial shift of 3.5 mm. Division of the posterior cruciate allows a posterior shift of 13 mm with greater motion of the lateral tibial plateau. *Note:* The medial and lateral plateaus were pulled in isolation equally with 3 Kg, either anteriorly or posteriorly

a true valgus injury. Only minimal loss of stability occurs if the medial capsular ligament and the posteromedial capsule are divided before cutting the medial ligament. If the medial ligament is injured, the posteromedial capsule acts as an important stabilizer. After severing all the medial components, however, both cruciate ligaments act as valgus stabilizers. According to the anatomic arrangement, the posterior cruciate should tear before the anterior in a valgus force. In practice, however, associated tears of the anterior cruciate ligament caused by additional external rotation are more frequent than injuries of the posterior curiate ligament. If the cruciate ligaments are intact, the valgus instability is decreased by internal rotation and increased by external rotation. The unloading of the posterior components during slight knee flexion increases the laxity of the normal as well as the injured knee [6].

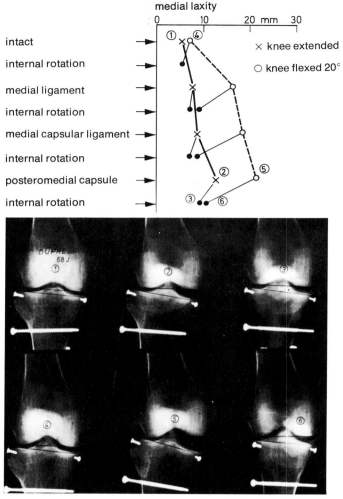

Fig. 6. Valgus instability with successive section of medial ligament, medial capsular band, and posteromedial capsule. X-rays were taken in neutral position and internal rotation of the lower leg, in full extension and with some flexion. Varus load 6 Kg. Instability is increased with some degree of knee flexion. However, even with full extension, medial opening increases, dependent upon the degree of the medial lesion. The knee joint becomes stabilized in all positions with internal rotation (3 in contrast to 2 in fully extended knee, 6 compared to 5 with some degree of knee flexion). The numbers of the X-ray series correspond to those in the diagram

Varus Instability

The lateral capsular ligamentous apparatus acts on varus stress in a fashion similar to the medial on valgus. With a pure varus trauma, the lateral ligaments, lateral capsular ligaments, and posterolateral capsule are also damaged in succession. The popliteus and biceps tendons are involved as well. An increase in flexion accentuates the varus laxity (Fig. 7) and this is decreased by internal rotation and increased by external rotation.

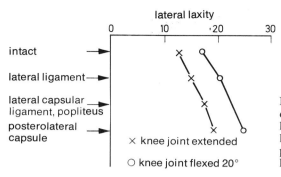

Fig. 7. Varus instability. Some degree of knee flexion increases the lateral laxity during all stages of lateral lesions, resembling the same process observed with the medial ligament

Technique for Examining Collateral Instability

Collateral ligament tension is decreased in slight knee flexion as compared to full extension. In both positions, however, the degree of instability increases corresponding to the degree of damage. Both medial and lateral ligaments should be examined in extension and slight flexion and compared with the findings in the uninjured knee (Figs. 6 and 7). It is important to note any degree of external rotation.

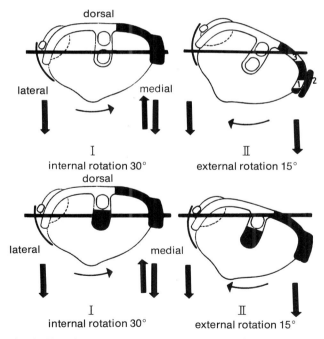

Fig. 8. Test for external rotation instability (Slocum and Larson). The anterior drawer test is carried out with the lower leg rotated in 2 positions (I and II). In position I, with internal rotation of the lower leg, the pull on the medial tibial plateau is neutralized. The anterior drawer sign then is positive only if there is instability of the posterolateral structures. In position II with lesions of the medial capsular ligamentous apparatus (upper right, sequence in external rotation trauma 1−2−3) only an increase of the external rotation is possible. A genuine rotation drawer sign can be produced only with an additional injury of the anterior cruciate ligament

Rotational Instability

The center of rotation of the normal knee lies within the medial femoral condyle next to the tibial eminence [18, 19]. This is true for both internal and external rotation. It is secured by the entire capsular ligamentous apparatus. Because of the medial position of this pivotal point, the lateral ligamentous capsular structures and the lateral tibial plateau have a greater range of motion during rotation than do the medial ligamentous capsular structures and the medial plateau. The degree of rotation varies from person to person. With 90° of flexion it can reach 90° [17]. The majority of this movement is external rotation and this is more by the posterior movement of the lateral than the anterior motion of the medial tibial plateau.

After ligament injury the center of rotation can change. Slocum and Larson [18] described a test for determining anteromedial rotatory instability (Fig. 8). This test is a modification of the anterior drawer sign. The anterior drawer is elicited with the foot in 30° of internal rotation (position 1). In this position posterolateral capsule and posterior cruciate ligaments prevent an anterior drawer even in the presence of a severed medial collateral and anterior cruciate.

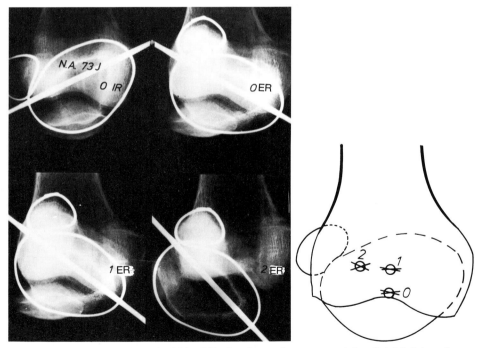

Fig. 9. X-rays of right knee in 90° of flexion from above toward the tibial joint surface. Wires mark the outline of the tibia and fibula. The transverse axis of the tibia is marked by a Steinmann pin. 0 normal knee; 1 division of medial ligamentous structures; 2 medial ligament division plus division anterior cruciate ligament; IR internal rotation, ER external rotation. The various centers during rotation are marked in the diagram. The centre moves only minimally in injuries of the medial capsular apparatus. A greater lateral shift occurs after division of the anterior cruciate ligament

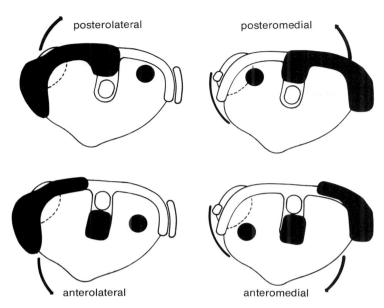

posterolateral   posteromedial

anterolateral   anteromedial

Fig. 10. The four different complex instabilities, according to Nicholas (top view of the right tibial joint surface). Dark black circle — center of rotation; dark surfaces — damaged ligamentous structures

In contrast, when the foot is rotated 15° externally (position 2), the anterior drawer sign reveals the anterior instability associated with the medial capsular ligamentous structures. The mediotibial plateau is moved increasingly forward depending upon the extent of the external rotational trauma, i.e., the sequence of medial capsular ligament, medial ligament, posterior medial capsule, and anterior cruciate ligament. According to Slocum and Larson this is the most sensitive test for anteromedial instability and the only one capable of revealing an isolated tear of the medial capsular ligament in external rotation forces since valgus stability remains intact. One should not be misled by this test. As long as the anterior cruciate ligament is intact, one is dealing with only increased external rotation of the mediotibial plateau around almost the same center of rotation as in the intact knee (Figs. 9 and 10). A significant lateral shift of the rotatory axis and a strongly positive drawer sign is observed only after division of the anterior cruciate ligament. It is then relatively unimportant whether the leg is maintained in a normal position or rotated externally since it rotates externally on its own, producing the rotational drawer syndrome. With forced internal rotation, however, the anterior drawer sign may be prevented because of the stability of the lateral tibial plateau and the posterolateral capsular structures (position 1).

Complex Instabilities

According to Nicholas, all instances in which collateral laxities are combined with a positive rotation drawer are termed complex instabilities. These are the

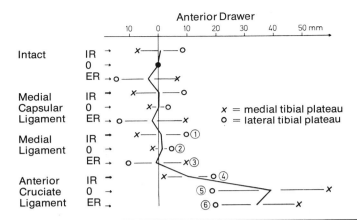

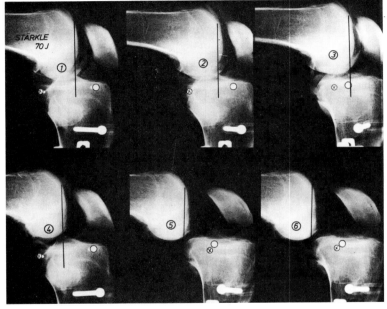

Fig. 11. This diagram shows the development of anteromedial complex instability caused by the serial section of the medial capsular ligament structures including the posteromedial capsule and the anterior cruciate ligament. An anterior force of 3 Kg was applied to the medial and lateral side of the tibia, allowing an internal, external, or neutral forward force. Internal rotation was 20°. External rotation similar, in the neutral position the tibia was not fixed and drawn straightforwardly. The anterior shift of the medial (⊗) and lateral (○) tibial plateaus is marked separately. The midposition of the tibia shifts only after the anterior cruciate ligament is divided. The positive anterior drawer sign (specimens 5 & 6) can be reduced by internal rotation of the tibia (specimen 4). The medial tibial plateau shows only a small degree of anterior shift with division of the medial ligament structures

result of extensive ligamentous tears. The common anteromedial complex instability is differentiated from the less common posteromedial, anterolateral, and posterolateral complexes [17] (Fig. 10). A complex instability is characterized by the following: noticeable shift of the rotatory axis, varus or valgus instability, positive anterior or posterior drawer, and by the fact that the rotation drawer can be stabilized to a considerable degree by counterrotation of the tibia. We were able to demonstrate various types of complex instabilities experimentally.

Review

The following facts have been established:

1. Knee flexion occurs in accordance with the laws of planar kinematics of a crossed four-jointed chain (four-bar linkage) that can be derived geometrically from the anatomic arrangement of the cruciate ligaments.
2. The axis of motion of knee flexion corresponds to the point of intersection of cruciate ligaments. During flexion it shifts from anterior to posterior.
3. The contours of the joints, the lateral ligaments, the contact points, and the centers of curvature are secondary to the kinematics of the cruciate ligament.
4. The capsular ligamentous system is as important for passive stability as the four main ligaments.
5. Loss of stability following an isolated anterior cruciate ligament lesion is minimal.
6. Various differences become obvious when testing for varus or valgus instability in full extension or slight flexion of the knee joint.
7. All varus and valgus instabilities with the laxity greater than 25 mm indicate a cruciate ligament tear.
8. With anteromedial complex instability the valgus position cannot be stabilized even with complete extension and internal rotation.
9. A significant shift of the center of rotation of the tibia occurs only with an associated lesion of a cruciate ligament.
10. No positive anterior or posterior gliding instability can be demonstrated without a lesion of the corresponding cruciate ligament and of at least one lateral ligament.
11. The medial rotatory instability described by Slocum and Larson, with an intact anterior cruciate ligament and a damaged medial ligament apparatus, represents an increased external rotation of the mediotibial plateau but not a genuine anterior gliding. With an additional lesion of the anterior cruciate ligament and a positive anterior glide a spontaneous rotation is present.
12. Counterrotation of the lower leg considerably stabilizes the various drawer signs for complex instabilities.

References

1. Brantigan, O. C., Voshell, A. F.: The mechanics of the ligaments and menisci of the knee joint. J. Bone Jt. Surg. **23**, 44 (1941)
2. Burri, C., Helbing, G., Rüter, A.: Die Behandlung der posttraumatischen Bandinstabilität am Kniegelenk. Orthopäde **3**, 184 (1974)

3. Castaing, J., Burdin, Ph., Mongin, M.: Les conditions de la stabilité passive du genou. Rev. Chir. Orthop. **58,** 34, Suppl. (1972)
4. Engin, A. E., Korde, M. S.: Biomechanics of normal and abnormal knee joint. J. Biomechanics **7,** 325 (1974)
5. Fick, R.: Handbuch der Anatomie und Mechanik der Gelenke. Jena: Fischer 1911.
6. Hönigschmied, J.: Leichenexperimente über die Zerreißung der Bänder im Kniegelenk. Dtsch. Z. Chir. **36,** 587 (1893)
7. Hughston, J. C.: Knee ligament injury in athletes. J. med. Ass. Ala. **36,** 243 (1966)
8. Hughston, J. C., Eilers, A. F.: The role of the posterior obbique ligament in repairs of acute medial (collateral) ligament tears of the knee. J. Bone Jt. Surg. **55 A,** 923 (1973)
9. Huson, A.: Biomechanische Probleme des Kniegelenkes. Orthopäde **3,** 119 (1974)
10. Kaplan, E. B.: Some aspects of functional anatomy of the human knee joint. Clin. Orthop. **23,** 18 (1962)
11. Kennedy, J. C., Fowler, J. P.: Medial and anterior instability of the knee – an anatomical and clinical study using stress machines. J. Bone Jt. Surg. **53 A,** 1257 (1971)
12. Kennedy, J. C., Grainger, R. W.: The posterior cruciate ligament. J. Trauma **7,** 367 (1967)
13. Langa, G. S.: Experimental observations and interpretations on the relationship between the morphology and function of the human knee joint. Acta anat. Basel, **55,** 16 (1963)
14. Liljedahl, S. O., Lindvall, N., Wetterfors, J.: Early diagnosis and treatment of acute ruptures of the anterior cruciate ligament. J. Bone Jt. Surg. **47 A,** 1503 (1965)
15. Menschik, A.: Mechanik des Kniegelenkes, 1. Teil. Z. Orthop. **112,** 481 (1974)
16. Meyer, H.: Die Mechanik des Kniegelenkes. Arch. Anat. Physiol. wiss. Med. (Müller's Archiv) 497 (1853)
17. Nicholas, J. A.: The five-one reconstruction for antero-medial instability of the knee. J. Bone Jt. Surg. **55 A,** 899 (1973)
18. Slocum, D. B., Larson, R. L.: Rotatory instability of the knee. J. Bone Jt. Surg. **50 A,** 211 (1968)
19. Steindler, A.: The mechanical analysis of the knee joint. In: Thomas C. C., Ed.: Kinesiology of the human body. pp. 330–340. Springfield/Ill.: Ch. C. Thomas 1955
20. Strasser, H.: Lehrbuch der Muskel- und Gelenkmechanik, Bd. III. Berlin: Springer 1917

Translation from the German: Biomechanik und Pathophysiologie des Kniebandapparates. In: Bandverletzungen am Knie, 3. Reisensburger Workshop zur klinischen Unfallchirurgie, edited by C. Burri and A. Rüter. In: Hefte zur Unfallheilkunde, Vol. 125 (1975). © Springer-Verlag 1975.

The Pathophysiology of Damage to Articular Cartilage

H. Cotta and W. Puhl

In discussing the pathophysiology of damage to articular cartilage in the knee joint, we shall consider the etiologic factors and pathogenetic mechanisms that can account for damage to a joint surface with a previously healthy bony base and cartilaginous covering.

Starting with different clinical situations we shall consider how cartilage damage is caused. If we succeed in bridging gaps in our knowledge of the pathogenetic chain between the clinical situation responsible and the resulting cartilage damage, we shall also learn something about therapeutic requirements.

Essential knowledge of the biology and physiology of the knee joint must first be reviewed. This will help us not only to appraise the extent to which the joint can compensate for various harmful influences, but also to consider what a healthy joint can stand, short of decompensation, and what reactions are to be expected when damage occurs.

Cartilage Architecture

Morphologic examination of articular cartilage reveals three constituents:
1. Collagen
2. Cartilage Cells
3. A largely amorphous basal ground substance in which the above-named elements are embedded.

The work of Benninghof [4] still contributes to an understanding of collagen structure. Near the joint surface the collagen fibers run tangentially, then they curve down obliquely through the cartilage, finally they reach the zone of calcified cartilage perpendicularly. The cells are correspondingly arranged. The superficial ones have their long axis parallel to the joint surface. In the next zone of cartilage growth the cells are more rounded and often lie in pairs. Near the subchondral bone their arrangement becomes columnar. In healthy adult cartilage collagen predominates near the surface and matrix predominates more deeply.

The chondrocyte synthesizes both the matrix and the collagen. The matrix has a uniform composition and a related water-binding capacity that guarantee the mechanical properties of cartilage. It contains negatively charged polysaccharide molecules known as glycosaminoglycans (GAG), (also called mucopolysaccharides). The most important are chondroitin-4-sulfate, chondroitin-6-sulfate, and keratin sulfate. As these are bound to protein the term proteoglycans is applied. The synthesis of chondroitin sulfates can be followed by incorporating radioactive sulfur. The proteoglycans make up most of the cartilage matrix and form a molecular microporous sponge, originally called a gel because of its mechanics. The glycosaminoglycans are synthesized by the chondrocytes. The synthesis is controlled by enzyme systems in the membranes of the cell organelles [39]. Degradative and synthesizing reactions continually run parallel. The half-life of the glycosaminoglycans is reported to be between several days and a few months [49].

Chondrocytes contain a number of lysosomal enzymes capable of breaking down matrix proteoglycan. Cathespsin D seems to be particularly important in this respect [1, 9, 25]. Proteoglycan can also be broken down by leukocyte enzymes at a neutral pH and by enzymes derived from rheumatic pannus [42, 74, 78, 79]. It seems significant that hyaluronidase can also break down proteoglycans [5].

The chondrocyte synthesizes procollagen which is made up of 3 polypeptide chains in parallel spirals. Once secreted, the procollagen is enzymatically cleaved to form the collagen fibril whose half-life is several months. The collagen imparts tensile strength to articular cartilage. According to investigations by Curtis and Klein [16, 17] proteolytic enzymes from chondrocytes cannot break down collagen in articular cartilage when the pH is within physiologic limits. During wound healing, however, it may be that special enzyme systems affect the denaturation of the collagen, hence its vulnerability to attack by enzymes [67]. It is also relevant to the pathophysiology of cartilage damage that a collagenase has been identified in granulocytes [45] and that increased collagen changes in arthrosis experimentally induced in animals have been related to degradative and synthesizing enzyme reactions [69].

Physical Properties of Cartilage

Healthy cartilage exhibits a characteristic mechanical behavior. A force applied to an articular surface immediately produces deformity in accordance with the elasticity of the tissue. Continuation of the pressure causes increasing deformity because fluid leaves the cartilage matrix in the area most under pressure and passes into less affected areas. The final deformity depends on the force acting, the osmotic pressure of the cartilage, the elasticity of its collagen, and the permeability of its matrix.

The resistance of cartilage to pressure is directly related to the glycosaminoglycan content of its matrix, the higher the glycosaminoglycan content, the less easily the tissue is deformed. The tensile strength of cartilage depends on its richness in collagen fibers. Resistance to tensile stress is greatest in the tangential zone.

Reaction of Cartilage to Physiologic Stress

The pattern of the morphologic structure of articular cartilage is not the same, quantitatively and qualitatively, in every case. On the contrary, by appropriate structural alterations, it reacts to changes in the mechanical demands made on it. Adaptation of this kind (one could call it the result of training) has been demonstrated in our investigations:

Femoral condyles of rabbit embryos have cells lying free beneath or on the articular surface devoid of any collagen. Histologic sections do not show the typical cartilage architecture well known to us from the text books. On the contrary, the tissue is richly cellular, is not differentiated into zones, and does not have a smooth surface. With increasing postnatal mechanical stress the articular surfaces progressively become smoother and the histologic picture increasingly becomes one of division into typical zones. An extensive study of human knee joints has produced similar findings [57, 59, 67].

Superficial cartilage cells can be seen in the articular surfaces of the still slightly loaded femoral condyles of neonates and small children. Increasing the loading leads to the superimposition of collagen structures, these are delicate at first. By further collagen synthesis the chondrocytes bury themselves until none can be seen near the surface. In their place are seen linear gradations produced by collagen bundles.

The loading to which articular surfaces are subjected varies enormously, both from one joint to another and in the same joint. This leads to corresponding structural differences. The surfaces of the weight-bearing areas of femoral condyles reveal only collagen bundles, but superficial cells are still seen on the posterior parts of the condyles. Other such differences [59] will be dealt with later when joint damage after meniscectomy is discussed.

Morphologic studies of articular cartilage demonstrate histologic responses to mechanical demands. Changes in demand evidently induce altered cell responses which affect the synthesis of collagen and cartilage matrix. With regard to the pathophysiology of knee damage, this means that suddenly increased demands can cause decompensation, hence the therapeutic aim of always giving articular cartilage time to adapt.

Nutrition of Articular Cartilage

The maintenance of normal structure, chemistry, and mechanics in cartilage means uninterrupted synthesis by chondrocytes. The nutrients which these cells

need to provide energy and to allow for necessary metabolic changes can be obtained by two routes:
1. via the vessels in the joint capsule
2. via the vessels in the subchondral bone.
Nutrient supply via the vessels in the subchondral bone is possible only in growing individuals with open epiphyseal plates [38, 50].

The sole route by which nutrients and oxygen are supplied to the articular cartilage in the fully grown, and an additional route in the still growing, is the vascular network of the joint capsule. Changes in this are, therefore, of prime importance in the pathophysiology of articular cartilage.

The synovial membrane of the joint capsule contains actively secreting and absorbing connective tissue cells. The capillaries within the synovial villi are arranged in loops [43, 44]. Raised pressure in the arterial limb causes filtration changes in the neighboring area. Substances are reabsorbed into the venous limb when the osmotic pressure in surrounding tissue exceeds the intravascular pressure.

This seemingly clear picture has been amended and amplified by our electron-microscopic investigations [10, 11, 13, 15, 19]. Cotta showed by electron microscopy that the capillary wall cannot be regarded as a simple semipermeable membrane. Instead, it is an unbroken tube made up of overlapping endothelial cells surrounded by an exceptionally thin basement membrane. Pericytes outside the basement membrane embrace the capillary wall. According to these morphologic findings, the transport of substances from the blood vascular system to the synovioctyes cannot be only by diffusion, filtration, and osmosis. In addition, the involvement of mechanisms permitting selective transport by the capillary endothelium must be assumed. Damage to capsular capillaries is, therefore, bound to have serious effects on joint nutrition since it restricts the transport of nutrients. This is an important reason why arthrosis develops after inflammatory and traumatic capsular changes. We shall consider this later.

However, the intracapsular transport of nutrients depends not only on the biologic performance of the capillary endothelium but also, as a physical phenomenon, on changes in the concentration and molecule size of the substance diffused and on the character of their diffusion pathway. The significance of the diffusion pathway has been alluded to by Cotta [11, 12, 13] and Cotta and Dettmer [15]. It is of interest in relation to the reduced compensatory potential of joints in old age, when the subsynovial layer becomes thicker and more extensive [70]. The capillary network thus moves further away from the capsular surface and substances from the bloodstream must traverse greater distances to reach the synoviocytes, joint cavity, and cartilage. The same applies to the transport of the end products of metabolism away from the cartilage and joint capsule.

The function of the joint capsule in lubrication of the joint is another important subject. The synoviocytes synthesize hyaluronic acid, and the extent to which this is polymerized determines the viscosity of the synovial fluid. As well as the hyaluronic acid molecules the protein molecules bound to them are the products of active synthesis by the synoviocytes. Other constituents of the synovial fluid such as glucose, electrolytes, and perhaps low molecular proteins, reach the joint cavity by diffusion from the intravascular space.

The cellular constituents of the synovia are almost exclusively leukocytes, of which there are normally fewer than 200 per mm. Lymphocytes and monocytoid cells are also seen. Inflammation produces cell counts of up to 200,000 per mm^3. This is another important point, the pathogenetic significance of which has been discussed by Greiling [29].

An important prerequisite for the flow of nutrients from joint capsule to articular cartilage (substrate transport in the synovia) is joint movement, which results in thorough mixing of the synovia. Movement also favors the diffusion of lactate (a breakdown product of cartilage metabolism) from the articular surface to the capsule.

Transport of substances in the articular cartilage itself is by diffusion. Variations in pressure on the articular surfaces during physiologic loading of the joint help by having a pumping effect. The microporous molecular sponge of proteoglycans allows substances with molecular weights of up to a few hundred to diffuse freely through its pores. Sugar and amino acids are examples. The tissue is, however, impervious to substances with molecular weights of more than 70.000 to 80.000 such as hyaluronic acid.

Pressure on a joint surface forces synovial fluid outward into the joint cavity and causes a flow of fluid and matrix in the cartilage into areas under less pressure.

When the pressure on the joint surface is removed, fluid flows back into the previously compressed cartilage. Scandinavian authors [40, 41] have demonstrated how joint function affects articular cartilage. Pressure change appeared to be important. Maroudas et al. [50] ascribed an invariably subsidiary role to the pump effect; mere movement of the fluid close to the cartilage was shown to increase the penetration of substances.

To sum up, it may be said that a normal blood supply, normal functioning of the capsular capillaries, an unimpeded intracapsular diffusion path, and continual movement of the synovial fluid are essential conditions for the exchange of substances between the intravascular space and articular cartilage.

Changes in Articular Cartilage With Aging

The impaired compensation potential of the joints of elderly and old people that is repeatedly observed in clinical work must be largely related to the changes in the joint capsule already mentioned. The following are not found in healthy cartilage in the adult: decreased number of cells [73], change in thickness of non-calcified cartilage [53], anomalies of tissue water content [46], changes in tissue elasticity [72], and significant variations in total glycosaminoglycan content [2]. Only a change in the relative proportions of keratan sulfate and chondroitin sulfate is observed between the third and fourth decades [74]. In addition the oxygen uptake of cartilage may decrease with aging.

Immobilization and Dystrophic Changes in Articular Cartilage

Immobilization of the knee joint causes, initially, a distinct reduction in the supply of blood to the joint capsule [28]. The resulting reduction in the supply of oxygen and nutrients in the articular cartilage can reach critical levels. Irreversible deposition of connective tissue in the joint capsule can also hinder the access of nutrients to the joint cavity and cartilage. Without thorough mixing of the synovia by joint movement, waste products of metabolism accumulate on the surface of the cartilage and nutrients needed by the cartilage accumulate on the capsule. The amount of lactate reaching the synoviocytes from the cartilage is reduced, and so hyaluronic acid production is diminished. By causing cartilage cell dystrophy, joint immobilization can, therefore, initiate an arthritic process [36, 51, 52, 54, 57, 58].

When the knee joint is immobilized its articular surfaces are held together under the pressure produced by the pull of muscles and any static loading there may be. In experimental studies in animals, Refior [68] showed that the highest pressures used led to regressive changes, with loss of cartilage matrix and exposure of collagen. Increasing disintegration of the articular cartilage was demonstrated by morphological and histochemical investigations.

Walcher and Stürz [76] found that pressure on immobilized joints in rabbits caused progressive loss of articular cartilage right down to the underlying bone.

By scanning electron microscopy we observed that prolonged immobilization without the application of pressure causes necrosis of chondrocytes in articular cartilage [14, 57, 67]. The articular surfaces show depressions corresponding in form, size and arrangement to chondrocytes; openings in the articular cartilage may be observed in these areas. In 1964 Ali [1] showed that intracellular enzymes can break down the surrounding cartilage matrix. The explanation of our findings must be that dystrophic cartilage cells die and release enzymes which destroy the surrounding cartilage matrix, and, if the cells are superficial, open up the articular surface.

The findings demonstrate the danger to cartilage that is associated with immobilization. The cartilage changes may be explained by dystrophy, by direct cell damage caused by pressure, and in some measure by changes in synthesis by chondrocytes, all in consequence of altered joint mechanics.

Immobilization with only physiologic pressure does not invariably cause macroscopically recognizable articular cartilage damage. After several years children with postencephalitic fixed knee joint extension have been found to have radiologically recognizable flattening of the femoral condyles without macroscopically recognizable damage to the condylar cartilage.

The knee is a joint which is often immobilized in extension. Hackenbroch has investigated the possible harmful effects by means of experiments using animals

[31, 32, 33]. He found that simple traction caused synovitis and histologically discernible degenerative changes in cartilage. That minor stresses on articular surfaces can hasten degeneration of their cartilage has often been emphasized [36, 54]. The important point is that synovitis can develop during joint traction and, by causing scarring, can lead to a lasting reduction in nutrient supply. With acute synovitis there is also the possibility of enzymatic damage to cartilage.

Joint Effusion and its Dystrophic Effects on Articular Cartilage

Effusion into the knee joint occurs in a variety of clinical situations. Serous effusion caused by nonspecific inflammation of the joint capsule will be considered separately from septic effusion and hemarthrosis. Serous effusions can occur with inflammation in the neighborhood of a joint, with gout, with articular manifestations of allergic states (as may be the case in postinfective rheumatoid arthritis), as well as after injury to the joint capsule. They can follow damage to articular cartilage and can result from damage to joint capsule capillaries, their possible cause in diseases of metabolism such as diabetes mellitus. The dangers to articular cartilage in all these cases are as follows:

1. By stretching the joint capsule the intraarticular effusion compresses the capsular capillaries. The resulting reduction in blood flow restricts the exchange of substances between the intravascular space and the cartilage. Consequential deposition of connective tissue in the joint capsule further interferes with nutrient supply. Furthermore, the increase in volume of the intraarticular fluid is a hindrance to the exchange of substances between the joint capsule and the articular cartilage. The increased volume of the intraarticular space also results in a relative reduction in lactate content. This is likely to restrict production of hyaluronic acid by the synoviocytes with the result that joint lubrication is impaired.

2. Synovitis causes increased entry of leukocytes into the joint space and production of lysosomal enzymes in the joint capsule. Enzymatic destruction of cartilage can result.

3. Large effusions cause stretching of ligaments thereby making joints less stable. This exposes the articular cartilage to the danger of unphysiologic stresses.

Serous effusions in rheumatoid arthritis in children and adults and in psoriatic arthritis require separate consideration. The destruction of articular cartilage in these diseases is caused mainly by enzymes from the joint capsule, rheumatic pannus, and granulocytes which have entered the joint (Fig. 1).

Hemarthrosis and Articular Cartilage Damage

Intraarticular hemorrhage, whether after trauma or in association with hemophilia, particularly endangers articular cartilage. In animals damage to articular

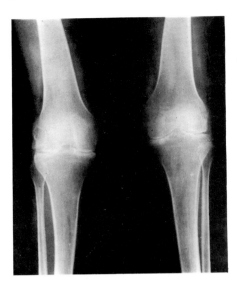

Fig. 1. Polyarthritis. Both knees fully involved. Typical end result of predominately enzymatic cartilage destruction

cartilage has been produced experimentally by only a few injections of an animal's own blood. Immobilization at the same time definitely increased the damage [23, 61, 66].

Possible ways in which hemarthrosis can damage articular cartilage in addition to those already attributed to effusions, are as follows:

1. The pronounced synovitis that occurs with hemarthrosis increases the length and density of the intracapsular transit path, thus reducing the flow of substrate between capsular capillaries and articular cartilage. Deposits of scar tissue in the joint capsule are particularly pronounced (Fig. 2).

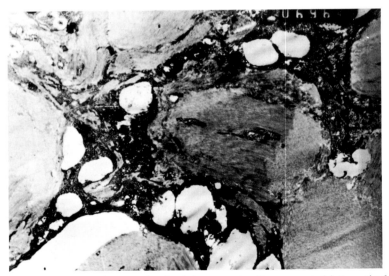

Fig. 2. Electron micrograph of a joint capsule after repeated intraarticular hemorrhage. Predominance of extensive collagen bundles (intracapsular scarring). Normal cell structures cannot be recognized. The intracapsular diffusion path is obstructed

2. Enzymes from the blood serum and leukocytes cause enzymatic destruction of superficial cartilage layers.

Hemarthrosis is, therefore, associated with an acute risk of enzymatic and dystrophic cartilage damage. It leaves a risk of chronic dystrophic damage.

Septic arthritis causes severe and rapid destruction of articular cartilage. The enzymes responsible come mainly from polymorphonuclear granulocytes [8, 34, 35, 37, 75, 79]. Using the scanning electron microscope to study articular cartilage after recurrent effusions, we have observed superficial lesions attributable to the localized action of granulocytic enzymes [56].

In summary, the two pathways leading to cartilage damage are insufficient cartilage nutrition resulting in dystrophic changes and direct enzymatic destruction.

Articular Cartilage and Injury

Fractures: Fractures near the knee joint can lead to cartilage damage by several of the mechanisms already discussed. Dystrophic damage can be caused by impairment of the joint capsule's arterial blood supply or venous return, and can result from immobilization either in plaster of Paris or by extension. Effusion into the knee joint during immobilization can also cause trophic or enzymatic damage to cartilage, and may itself be caused by interference with the circulation.

Isolated cartilage injury means either the shearing off of a thin layer of cartilage from the joint surface or the rupturing and consequent fissuring of the articular cartilage. The latter is probably common with contusions of the knee joint, and is often undetected at first radiological examination. Whatever the nature and mechanism of the first disruption or destruction of the joint surface, it causes two fundamentally different reactions in the articular cartilage. These are regeneration and degeneration, and their relative extents determine the subsequent fate of the joint [62, 65].

First, superficial cells of the articular cartilage produce replacement tissue rich in cells and collagen. In experiments in animals this has been proved capable of filling a 0.5 mm wide defect. The initially polygonal cells, resembling fibrocytes, become more and more rounded. The cells in the deeper zones become surrounded by lacunae, like those in fibrocartilage and hyaline cartilage. With the production of cartilage matrix, collagen structures stand out more clearly in the histological picture. After three months tissue that could be called fibrocartilage, or hyaline cartilage in some cases, has thus been formed. Animal studies have shown that the extent of tissue replacement depends on the age of the subject. The younger the animal, the greater the possibility for regeneration [20].

Degenerative processes are seen at the same time as these attempts to fill defects or seal openings in the joint surface. Chondrocytes in the neighborhood of fissures and in the margins of cartilage defects die, especially in the intermediate and deeper zones. The result is cell depopulation and reduction in tissue glycosaminoglycan content, revealed by hypochromasia. However, cell clusters like those seen in arthritic cartilage are also observed. These are closely packed collections of cells which expand peripherally by cell division while cells in the center die. Sulfur uptake increases [22, 47, 48] indicating increased synthesis of chondroitin sulfate, the principal glycosaminoglycan of cartilage.

Nevertheless, no real increase in cartilage has been observed (such an increase would allow the cells to move apart). On the contrary, the glycosaminoglycan content in the vicinity of the clusters is diminished. It must be concluded that the increase in synthesis coincides with a still greater increase in degradation. Figuratively speaking the clusters devour their mother tissue.

If the regenerative processes predominate, the cartilage injury can heal without clinical sequelae. If degenerative processes predominate, an arthrosis will result. However, investigations in animals have shown that drugs can curb the degenerative processes and promote the regenerative ones [22, 63, 64].

Intraarticular fractures involving the knee joint can cause cartilage damage in any of the ways already dealt with in discussing hemarthrosis. In addition, chondrocytes may be damaged by phagocytosing lipids that have entered the synovial fluid from bone. Cartilage in the fracture line is damaged in ways already described. Also, granulation tissue growing out from the subchondral bone can fill the fracture line up to the joint surface. With sufficient stress there can be metaplastic change into fibrocartilage [24, 71]. If an intraarticular fracture leaves a step in the joint surface, excessive mechanical strain can cause destruction of articular cartilage. This will be dealt with when chronic damage to articular cartilage is discussed.

Capsular Derangement: Injury confined to the joint capsule is common. Examples are contusion, twisting, and tearing. Tearing can cause further damage through intraarticular bleeding. Secondary scarring may remain after the highly vascular joint capsule has healed. Effects on capsular blood supply, and therefore, on the nutrition of the articular cartilage can be drastic (Fig. 3).

Capsular trauma, even without hemarthrosis, is often followed by recurrent nonsanguinous effusions. These indicate disturbed regulation of capsular elements engaged in secretion and absorption. Chronic recurrent synovitis and interference with capsular blood supply are often the cause. Recurrent knee joint effusions endanger articular cartilage. Nutritional and enzymatic damage and impaired joint lubrication can produce manifest arthrosis (Fig. 4).

At arthrotomy of such joints perhaps done for diagnostic reasons the cartilage surface can look unremarkable macroscopically or, at the most, only slightly damaged. Examination under the scanning electron microscope shows exposed collagen fibers, indicating considerable loss of cartilage matrix. As the collagen-rich tangential zone of the articular cartilage is subject to much less enzymatic destruction than the underlying proteoglycan-rich zone, frequent pennantlike

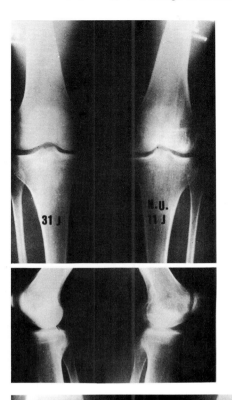

Fig. 3. Arthritis of left knee 11 years after dislocation. Causes of the damage are vascular sequelae, hemarthrosis, immobilization, and ligamentous laxity

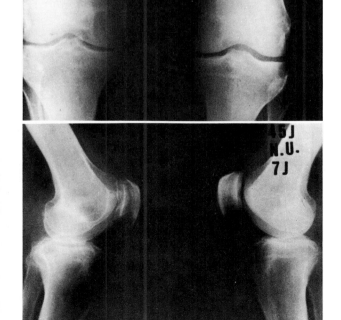

Fig. 4. Arthritis of right knee. Forty-five-year-old male. Seven years after severe contusion injury, subsequent recurrent effusions. Biopsy revealed chronic nonspecific synovitis. Comparison with the other knee demonstrates the gravity of the traumatic synovitis

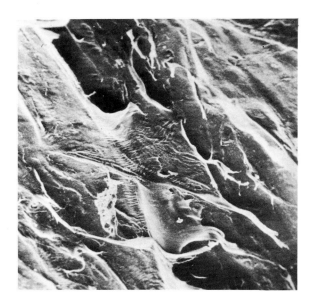

Fig. 5. Scanning electron micrograph of condylar surface of femur after recurrent effusions. Characteristic exposure of collagen structures (in the center) and pennant-shaped elevations of the collagen-rich, surface layer of the articular cartilage

elevations of the most superficial cartilage layers are seen (Fig. 5). Thus the danger with injury to the joint capsule is, at first, interference with cartilage nutrition and damage by hemarthrosis and then the development of a chronic recurrent synovitis which causes extensive nutritional and enzymatic cartilage damage.

Ligament Derangement: Injuries to ligaments can cause cartilage damage in the same ways as capsular injuries. In addition, permanent instability of a joint after ligamentous injury can interfere with the lubrication of its articular surfaces. Friedebold [27] speaks of functional incongruity. Clinical investigations have also led other authors to stress the harmful consequences of inadequate ligamentous control of the knee joint [6, 18].

Effects of Meniscectomy: Trauma causing meniscus damage can also injure articular cartilage. Regenerative and degenerative changes follow. We wish to emphasize the possibility of damage to articular cartilage after meniscectomy. The structure of articular cartilage on the tibial plateau directly under the meniscii differs from that of the cartilage not covered by the meniscii. Diversities in cartilage differentiation can be attributed to differences in mechanical demands [57, 59, 67]. When a meniscus is removed, the underlying articular cartilage is exposed to demands for which it was not built. Early unrestricted use of the joint can conceivably cause mechanical abrasion of the cartilage on the tibial plateau. Damage to articular cartilage so caused may account for some of the unsatisfactory late results after meniscectomy (Fig. 6). Hence the therapeutic need for gradual rehabilitation over a period of months, so as to give the cartilage tissue the opportunity to adapt to altered mechanical conditions.

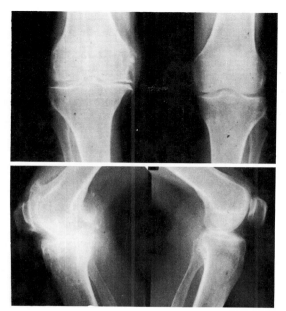

Fig. 6. Arthritis of right knee. Sixty-seven-year-old female. Thirty years after right medial meniscectomy. Left knee practically normal

Disproportionate Demands on Joints: Abnormal configuration of knee joint surfaces, either after intraarticular fractures or caused by faulty growth after epiphyseal damage or indeed congenital or acquired malalignment of the joint, can cause the demands made on articular cartilage to be so out of proportion to its ability to meet them that decompensation results. Whether excessive pressure interferes with synthesis by the chondrocytes, such that diminished production of proteoglycans leads to an alteration in the mechanical properties of cartilage and a reduction in its loading capacity, or whether disruption of the film of lubricant first causes splitting of the surface through dry friction, is difficult to decide in any given case. In principle, both mechanisms are possible. In all cases the first effects of cartilage wear and tear are fibrillation, roughening of the surface, and hypochromasia indicating a reduction in glycosaminoglycan content. It is interesting that in these cases it can be assumed that the cartilage had time to exhaust every possibility for adapting to heavy demands before the damage occurs. Increased loading occasions an increase in the thickness of articular cartilage (in the knee joint, e.g., the cartilage is naturally thicker than in a finger joint). Increase in thickness seems to be limited by joint nutrition, or, more precisely, by the intraarticular path attainable. Whether a mechanically desirable increase in articular cartilage can be fully attained, therefore, depends on the nutritional potential of the joint.

Mechanical destruction of cartilage can occur with physiologic stress on abnormal cartilage. This happens with ochoronosis and gout when the tissue is rendered more rigid by incrustation with uric acid crystals. Mechanical breaching of a joint surface under physiologic loading is also conceivable if joint

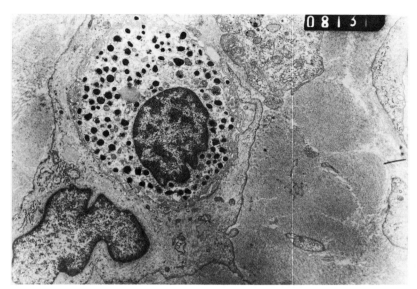

Fig. 7. Electron micrograph of knee joint capsule. Synovitis induced by posttraumatic articular cartilage damage. Extensive collagen bundles, these obstruct the intracapsular diffusion path. The cells near the center contain an excess of lysosomes, enzymes from these contribute to the synovitis and can damage the articular cartilage

lubrication is inadequate. This can happen with arthritis and in old people, in whose articular cartilage the degree of polymerization of hyaluronic acid is diminished [7].

Excessive loading can occur with actual trauma and can be assumed to occur with congenital deformities and acquired loose bodies in joints.

In the area where articular cartilage is first destroyed, the congruity of the joint surfaces is no longer optimal, nor, therefore, is their lubrication. Further physiologic loading then causes more mechanical wear and tear. During the weight-bearing phase of movement, synovial membrane is forced under pressure into the primary defect. This happens to a much smaller extent during the succeeding non-weight-bearing phase of movement in the reverse direction. The result is asymmetric extension of the original damage to the joint surface.

Further mechanical wear and tear of the articular surface destroys chondrocytes. Hitherto cell-bound enzyme activity can now break down cartilage matrix and induce inflammatory changes in the joint capsule, causing joint capsule pain. Synovitis causes joint capsule scarring and edema; joint nutrition is thus impaired, because the intracapsular diffusion path is lengthened and obstructed (Fig. 7).

Further enzymatic destruction of cartilage results from the activation of previously inactive enzyme precursors, increased formation of lysosomes in the synoviocytes, and increased migration of leukocytes into the joint capsule and joint space. Mechanical destruction and enzymatic destruction of articular cartilage proceed in a vicious circle. The end result can be complete wearing away of cartilage and the exposure of subchondral bone.

References

1. Ali, S. Y.: The degradation of cartilage matrix by an intracellular protease. Biochem. J. **93**, 611 (1964)
2. Anderson, C. E., Ludowieg, J., Harper, H. A., Engleman, E. P.: The composition of the organic component of human articular cartilage. J. Bone Jt. Surg. **46 A,** 1176 (1964)
3. Bennett, G. A., Waine, H., Bauer, W.: Changes in the knee joint at various ages. The Commonwealth Fund Ltd. **III,** 1178 (1942)
4. Benninghoff, A.: Form und Bau der Gelenkknorpel in ihren Beziehungen zur Funktion. 2. Teil: Der Aufbau des Gelenkknorpels in seinen Beziehungen zur Funktion Z. wiss. Biol., Abt. B, Z. Zellforsch. **2,** 783 (1925)
5. Bollet, A. J., Bonner, W. M., Nance, J. L.: The presence of hyaluronidase in various mammalian tissues. J. biol. Chem. **238,** 10, 3522 (1963)
6. Bühler, A.: Die hohe Tibiaosteotomie in der Behandlung der Gonarthrose. Diss. Basel (1974)
7. Castor, C. W., Prince, R. K., Hazelton, M. J.: Hyaluronic acid in human synovial effusions; a sensitive indicator of altered connective tussue cell function during inflammation. Arthr. and Rheum. **9,** 738 (1966)
8. Caygill, I. C., Pitkeathly, D. V.: A study of β-acethylglucosaminase and acid phosphatase in pathological joint fluids. Ann. rheum. Dis. **25,** 137 (1966)
9. Chrisman, O. D., Fessel, J. M.: Enzymatic degradation of chondromuco protein by cell-free extracts of human cartilage. Surg. Forum **13,** 444 (1962)
10. Cotta, H.: Elektronenmikroskopische Untersuchungen am Bindegewebe der Gelenkkapsel. Verh. dtsch. orthop. Ges. **49,** Kongr. Zürich, 27, September 1961
11. Cotta, H.: Pathophysiologische Reaktionen der Gelenke. Verh. dtsch. orthop. Ges. **51,** 263 (1964)
12. Cotta, H.: Das Arthroseproblem unter Berücksichtigung neuer Ergebnisse der Bindegewebsforschung. Med. Klinik **60,** 1566 (1965)
13. Cotta, H.: Die Bedeutung der Gelenkkapsel für degenerative Gelenkerkrankungen unter Berücksichtigung elektronenoptischer Untersuchungen. 1. Gemeinschaftskongress Deutsch. orthop. Ges. und Societa Italiana di Orthopedia e Traumatologio, 27.–30. April 1966. Stuttgart: Ende 1968
14. Cotta, H.: Die Pathogenese der Gonarthrose. Z. Orthop. **111,** 490 (1973)
15. Cotta, H., Dettmer, N.: Ergebnisse der Bindegewebsforschung und ihre Bedeutung für Erkrankungen des Stütz- und Bewegungsapparates. Arch. orthop. Unfall-Chir. **52,** 217 (1960)
16. Curtiss, P. H., Klein, L.: Destruction of articular cartilage in septic arthritis. J. Bone Jt. Surg. **45 A,** I (1963)
17. Curtiss, P. H., Klein, L.: Destruction of articular cartilage in septic arthritis. J. Bone Jt. Surg. **47 A,** II (1965)
18. Debeyre, J., Artigou, J. M.: Les indications et les résultats de l'ostéotomie tibiale. Rev. Chir. orthop. **59,** 641 (1973)
19. Dettmer, N., Cotta, H.: Elektronenmikroskopische Untersuchungen über das Bindegewebe der Gelenkkapsel. II. Mitteilung: Die Capillaren der menschlichen Gelenkkapsel. Z. Orthop. **96,** 186 (1962)
20. Dustmann, H. O., Puhl, W.: Altersabhängige Heilungsmöglichkeiten von Knorpelwunden. Z. Orthop. − im Druck
21. Dustmann, H. O., Puhl, W., Krempien, B.: Das Phänomen der Cluster im Arthroseknorpel. Arch. orthop. Unfall-Chir. **79,** 321 (1974)
22. Dustmann, H. O., Puhl, W., Martin, K.: Der Einfluß intraarticulärer Arteparoninjektionen bei Arthrose − Tierexperimentelle Untersuchungen. Z. Orthop. **112,** 1188 (1974)
23. Dustmann, H. O., Puhl, W., Schulitz, K. P.: Knorpelveränderungen beim Hämarthros unter besonderer Berücksichtigung der Ruhigstellung. Arch. orthop. Unfall-Chir. **71,** 148 (1971)
24. Dustmann, H. O., Schulitz, K. P., Puhl, W.: Der Schienbeinkopfbruch als Präarthrose. Z. Orthop. **112,** 637 (1974)
25. Fessel, J. N., Chrisman, O. D.: Enzymatic degradation of chondromucoprotein by cell-free extracts of human cartilage. Arthr. and Rheum. **7,** 393 (1964)

26. Freeman, M. A. R.: Adult Articular Cartilage. Oxford: Alden & Mowbray Ltd. at the Alden Press 1973

27. Friedebold, G.: Die posttraumatische Arthrose. Hefte z. Unfallheilkunde **110,** 127 (1971)

28. Goerthler, K.: Grenzen und Möglichkeiten der Diagnostik entzündlicher Kniegelenkserkrankungen durch Punktion und Exzision. Z. Orthop. **92,** 275 (1959)

29. Greiling, H., Kisters, R., Engels, G.: Die Enzyme in der Synovialflüssigkeit und ihre pathophysiologische Bedeutung. Enzymologie **30,** 135 (1966)

30. Grillo, H. C., Gross, J.: Collagenolytic activity during mammalian wound repair. Develop. Biol. **15,** 300 (1967)

31. Hackenbroch, M. H.: Gelenkveränderungen unter dosierter Druckminderung im Tierversuch. Z. Orthop. **112,** 667 (1974 a)

32. Hackenbroch, M. H.: Biopolymere und Biomechanik von Bindegewebssystemen. 7. Wissenschaftliche Konferenz Deutscher Naturforscher und Ärzte. Berlin–Heidelberg–New-York: Springer 1974 b

33. Hackenbroch, M. H., Springer, H.-H.: Tierexperimentelle Untersuchungen zur Frage der Reversibilität destraktionsbedingter Gelenkveränderungen. Z. Orthop. **112,** 140 (1974)

34. Hamerman, D., Janis, R., Smith, C.: Cartilage matrix depletion by rheumatoid synovial calls in tissue culture. J. exp. Med. **126,** 1005 (1967)

35. Hammerman, D., Sandson, J., Schubert, M.: Biochemical events on joint disease. J. Chron. Dis. **16,** 835 (1963)

36. Harrison, M. H. M., Schajowicz, F., Trueta, J.: Osteoarthritis of the hip: A study of the nature and evolution of the disease. J. Bone Jt. Surg. **53 B,** 589 (1953)

37. Hirsch, J. G., Cohn, Z. A.: Leucocyte lysosomes. Cell-Bound Antibodies, **15** (1963)

38. Hodge, J., McKibbin, B.: The nutrition of mature and immature joint cartilage in rabbits. J. Bone Jt. Surg. **51 B,** 140 (1969)

39. Horwitz, A. Dorfman, A.: Subcellular sites for synthesis of chondromucoprotein of cartilage. J. Cell Biol. **38,** 258 (1968)

40. Ingelmark, B. E., Ekholm, R.: A study on variations in the thickness of articular cartilage in association with rest and periodic load. Upsala Läk-Fören. Forh. **53,** 61 (1948)

41. Ingelmark, B. E., Saaf, J.: Über die Ernährung des Gelenkknorpels. Acta Orthop. Scand. **17,** 303 (1948)

42. Janoff, A., Blondin, J.: Depletion of cartilage matrix by a neutral protease fraction of human leucocyte lysosomes. Proc. Soc. exp. Biol. (N. Y.) **135,** 302 (1970)

43. Lang, J.: Wie verändert sich die Gelenkinnenhaut im Laufe des Lebens? Die Biomorphose der Gelenkinnenhaut. Verh. dtsch. orthop. Ges. **46,** 126 (1959)

44. Lang, J.: Anatomische, funktionell wichtige Baumerkmale der Gelenkinnenhaut. Verh. dtsch. orthop. Ges. **46,** 323 (1959)

45. Lazarus, G. S., Daniels, J. R., Brown, R. S., Bladen, H. A., Fullmer, H. M.: Degradation of collagen by a human granulocyte collagenolytic system. J. Clin. Invest. **47,** 2622 (1968)

46. Linn, F. C., Sokoloff, L.: Movement and composition of interstitial fluid of cartilage. Arthr. and Rheum. **8,** 481 (1965)

47. Mankin, H. J., Lippiello, L.: The turnover of adult rabbit articular cartilage. J. Bone Jt. Surg. **51 A,** 1591 (1969)

48. Mankin, H. J., Lippiello, L.: Biochemical and metabolic abnormalities in articular cartilage from osteo-arthritic human hips. J. Bone Jt. Surg. **52 A,** 424 (1970)

49. Maroudas, A.: in Freeman, M. A. R. Adult Articular Cartilage. Oxford: Alden & Mowbray Ltd. at the Alden Press 1973

50. Maroudas, A., Bullough, P., Swanson, S. A. V., Freeman, M. A. R.: The permeability of articular cartilage. J. Bone Jt. Surg. **50 B,** 166 (1968)

51. Matthiass, A. H.: Die Reaktion der Gelenke auf Behandlungsmaßnahmen. Verh. dtsch. orthop. Ges. 51. Kongr. 335 (1965)

52. Matthiass, A. H., Glupe, J.: Immobilisation und Druckbelastung in ihrer Wirkung auf die Gelenke. Arch. orthop. Unfall-Chir. **60,** 380 (1966)

53. Meachim, G.: Effect of age on the thickness of adult articular cartilage at the shoulder joint. Ann rheim. Dis. **30,** 43 (1971)

54. Morscher, E.: Resultate der subkapitalen Keilosteotomie bei der Epiphyseolysis capitis femoris. Z. Orthop. **49,** 256 (1961)
55. Morscher, E.: Mikrotrauma und traumatische Knorpelschäden als Arthroseursache. Z. Unfallmed. Berufskrankh. **4** (1974)
56. Puhl, W.: Rasterelektronenmikroskopische Untersuchungen zur Frage früher Knorpelschädigungen durch leukocytäre Enzyme. Arch. orthop. Unfall-Chir. **70,** 87 (1971)
57. Puhl, W.: Die Mikromorphologie der Gelenkknorpeloberfläche — rasterelektronenmikroskopische Untersuchungen an normalen und pathologisch veränderten Gelenkflächen. Habilitationsschrift Heidelberg 1972
58. Puhl, W.: Die Alterung des Bindegewebes und ihr Einfluß auf den Haltungs- und Bewegungsapparat. Aktuelle Gerontologie **3,** 2. Stuttgart: Thieme 1973
59. Puhl, W.: Die Mikromorphologie gesunder Gelenkknorpeloberflächen. Z. Orthop. **112,** 262 (1974 a)
60. Puhl, W.: Die Osteochondritis dissecans des Kniegelenkes als Präarthrose. Z. Orthop. **112,** 634 (1974 b)
61. Puhl, W., Dustmann, H. O.: Der Einfluß intraartikulärer Trasylolinjektionen beim Hämarthros — Tierexperimentelle Untersuchungen. Z. Orthop. **110,** 42 (1972)
62. Puhl, W., Dustmann, H. O.: Die Reaktionen des Gelenkknorpels auf Verletzungen — Tierexperimentelle Untersuchungen. Z. Orth. **111,** 494 (1973)
63. Puhl, W., Dustmann, H. O.: Der Einfluß intraarticulärer Glukosamin-Injektionen bei Arthrose (im Druck)
64. Puhl, W., Dustmann, H. O.: Tierexperimentelle Untersuchungen zur Beeinflußbarkeit der Arthrose durch intramuskuläre Gabe von Arteparon (im Druck)
65. Puhl, W., Dustmann, H. O., Quosdorf, U.: Tierexperimentelle Untersuchungen zur Regeneration des Gelenkknorpels. Arch. orthop. Unfall-Chir. **74,** 352 (1973)
66. Puhl, W., Dustmann, H. O., Schulitz, K. P.: Knorpelveränderungen bei experimentellen Hämarthros. Z. Orthop. **109,** 3, 475 (1971)
67. Puhl, W., Iyer, V.: Sem observations on the structure of the articular cartilage surface in normal and pathological condition. Scanning Electron Microscopy 1973 (Part III). Proceedings of the Workshop an Scanning Electron Microscopy in pathology. IIT Research Institute. Chicago, Illinois 60616, U. S. A. — April 1973
68. Refior, H. J.: Tierexperimentelle Untersuchungen zum Verhalten der Mikroarchitektur des hyalinen Gelenkknorpels unter Druck-Belastung. Habil.-Schrift München 1973
69. Repo, R. U., Mitchell, N.: Collagen synthesis in mature articular cartilage of the rabbit. J. Bone Jt. Surg. **53 B,** 541 (1971)
70. Ruckes, J., Schuckmann, F.: Frankfurt, Z. Path. **72,** 243 (1962)
71. Schulitz, K. P., Dustmann, H. O., Puhl, W.: Die Entwicklung der posttraumatischen Arthrose am Beispiel des Schienbeinbruches. Arch. orthop. Unfall-Chir. **76,** 136 (1973)
72. Sokoloff, L.: Elasticity of aging cartilage. Fed. Proc. **25,** 1089 (1966)
73. Stockwell, R. A.: The cell density of human articular and costal cartilage. J. Anat. (Lond.) **101,** 753 (1967)
74. Stockwell, R. A.: Changes in the acid glycosaminoglycan content of the matrix of aging human articular cartilage. Ann. rheum. Dis. **29,** 509 (1970)
75. Sylven, B.: Cartilage and chondroitin sulphate. III. Chondroitin sulphate and inflammatory lesions of cartilage. J. Bone Jt. Surg. **30 A** (1948)
76. Walcher, K. Stürz, H.: Weitere Beobachtungen zur Frage der Regenerationsfähigkeit hyalinen Knorpels. Arch. Chir. **331,** 1 (1972)
77. Weissman, G.: Lysosomes and Joint Disease. Arthr. and Rheum., Vol. **9,** No. 6 (December 1966)
78. Weissman, G., Spilberg, J.: Breakdown of cartilage proteinpolysaccharide by lysosomes. Arth. and Rheum. **11,** 162 (1968)
79. Ziff, M., Gribetz, H. J., Lospalluto, J.: Effect of leucocyte and synovial membrane extracts on cartilage mucoprotein. J. Clin. Invest. **36,** 1 (1960)

Translation from the German: Pathophysiologie des Knorpelschadens. In: Knorpelschaden am Knie, 4. Reisensburger Workshop zur klinischen Unfallchirurgie, edited by C. Burri and A. Rüter. In: Hefte zur Unfallheilkunde, Vol. 127 (1976). © Springer-Verlag 1976.

The Reaction of Articular Cartilage to Pressure, Immobilization, and Distraction

H. J. Refior and M. H. Hackenbroch Jr.

Introduction

Not only biologic factors, but also the differing mechanical circumstances with which joints contend are important in the etiology of athrosis. Clinical observations as well as experimental studies in animals support this view. How far arthritic changes can be produced experimentally in animals by the prolonged action of mechanical influences on articular cartilage is the subject of the present investigations. The method has been to observe and evaluate the micromorphologic changes produced by measured compression and by measured distraction during immobilization.

Joint changes after compression and immobilization have been reported before [14, 17 etc.], but without detailing the early changes in hyaline articular cartilage and the behavior of the microarchitecture. Clinical relevance has seldom been clear.

Very little information is available about joint distraction used experimentally in animals. This adds to the interest of the present investigations, which were designed to contribute to the understanding of clinical observations after the therapeutic use of extension.

1. Experimental Compression and Immobilization

Trueta stated in 1956 that unphysiologic distribution of pressure within a joint causes degenerative changes beginning in the articular cartilage. The aim of the experiments now described was to determine the early changes induced in hyaline articular cartilage by measured compression during immobilization. The observations were made on the knee joint in the rabbit. The behavior of the different structural elements in cartilage was studied by a variety of methods and was documented. An attempt was also made to arrive at a morphologic definition of prearthrosis, a predominately clinical concept.

Materials and Methods

The investigations were carried out in 156 young fully grown rabbits weighing between 3000 and 4200 g.

The means of compression chosen was based on the principle of the tension device used by Greifensteiner and Charnley. It permits compression to be extraarticular. A modified form of the apparatus described by Crelin and Southwick was used. The knee joint was immobilized by external splinting of the hind limb with the knee flexed at an acute angle. Intravenous Nembutal anesthesia was used during the operative procedure (Fig. 1).

The spring force used in compression at the beginning of each experiment was 12 kp. The average drop in force during the experiments was 15–30%.

One advantage of the experimental method described was the almost complete immobilization obtained. Damage to articular cartilage after incomplete immobilization reported by other authors [6, 10] was thus avoided. Another advantage of using extraarticular compression was the avoidance of additional intraarticular damage, as might be expected from introducing a transarticular compression bolt [17].

The animals were divided into groups with postoperative investigation periods of either four or seven days, and two, three or four weeks. Control animals had only immobilization of one hind leg; their investigation periods were either two or four weeks. The animals were killed and both knee joints examined macroscopically. The left knee joint served as a control. Histological preparations were then stained by several methods, hamatoxilin and eosin, Van Gieson's, Goldner's method, or by histochemical staining combinations alcian blue, PAS or astra blue nuclear fast reduction.

In order to exclude artefacts, unfixed and glutaraldehyde fixed sections of articular cartilage were examined by direct light microscopy. The preparations

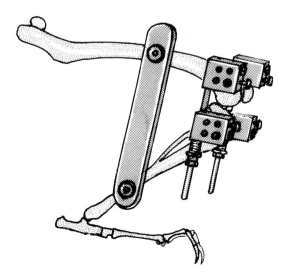

Fig. 1. Method used to immobilize and compress the knee joint in the rabbit

for examination by scanning electron microscopy were cleansed and then fixed for 3–4 h in a 3.5% buffered solution of glutaraldehyde. Rinsing was followed by freeze-drying. The preparations were then coated with carbon and gold and examined with the scanning electron microscope Stereoscan Mark IIA (Cambridge Instrument Company).

Results and Discussion

Direct light microscopy and scanning electron microscopy of intact articular surfaces from fully grown laboratory animals reveal two distinct patterns. Correspondingly different structural arrangements are described.

Both undulations running nearly parallel [3, 7, 11] and shallow, randomly arranged, round or ovoid surface depressions, giving the impression of a mesh-worklike structure, are observed [2, 7, 33]. Such surface patterns, described in human and many different animal preparations, were also seen on articular cartilage from the knees and the elbow joints of our rabbits (Fig. 2). It seems justifiable to assume that these structural patterns have a biologic significance.

As our studies confirm, the surface pattern of articular cartilage in the fully grown subject depends mainly on the fibers in the tangential zone. Similar appearances are seen beyond the cartilage contact areas if there is progressive loss of basic amorphous substance (Fig. 3).

According to theoretical analysis of stress distribution in articular cartilage [18] the surface pattern determined by the fibrillary structures is related to function.

After compression for only four days under the experimental conditions described, histological sections showed hypochromasia of the nuclei of the chondrocytes in the tangential and intermediate zones. Scanning electron microscopy

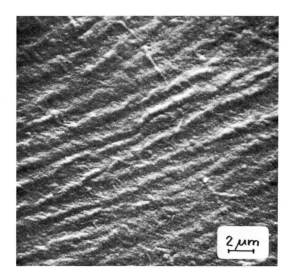

2 μm

Fig. 2. Nearly parallel array of undulations on the surface of healthy articular cartilage (× 5000)

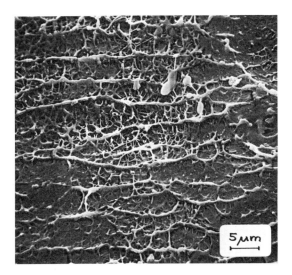

Fig. 3. Loss of basic substance reveals an orderly array of collagen fibril bundles connected by finer bundles ($\times$ 2200)

showed commencing exposure of fibrillary structures in the cartilage contact zones. However, surface patterns were still physiologic (Fig. 4).

Compression lasting seven days produced increasing surface changes in the cartilage zones. Especially on the tibial articular surfaces, loss of amorphous ground substance had increased, with more pronounced exposure of reticular fibrillary structures. The latter largely retained their orientation (Fig. 5).

Histological examination showed shrinking of cells in the tangential zone and increasingly numerous pyknotic nuclei. At the edge of the pressure area a deviation in orientation of rows of cells toward the periphery was not invariably seen in the radial zone (Fig. 6). These findings correlate with those of other authors [14, 17].

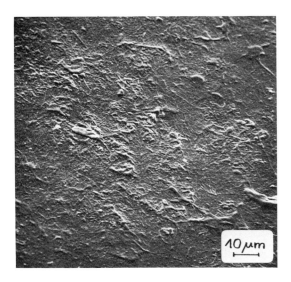

Fig. 4. Cartilage contact zone after four day experiment. Exposure of fiber structures is beginning ($\times$ 1000)

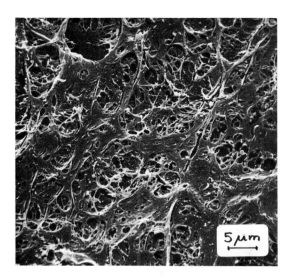

Fig. 5. Pressure center of cartilage contact zone after one week experiment. Exposure of fiber texture, still partly clouded with ground substance ($\times$ 2200)

Scanning electron microscopy (SEM) in the two-week experiments showed definite destructive changes in the articular cartilage surface. The main ones were the detachment of thin flakes or lamellae, together with tearing or rupturing of fibrillar structures. It was now hard to see an orderly arrangement, although a three-dimensional network of fibers was still recognizable. Histological examination showed a reduction in the number of cells in the tangential and intermediate zones, a change in the staining of ground substance, and some shrinking of chondrocytes in the radial zone. Rupturing and flaking were now seen in the tangential zone. Similar changes have been observed after experimentally induced hemarthrosis and immobilization [5].

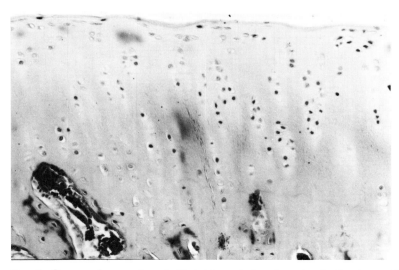

Fig. 6. One week experiment. Shrinking of chondrocytes in the tangential fiber zone, nuclei, and deviation of rows of cells in the radial zone (Goldner's stain, $\times$ 63)

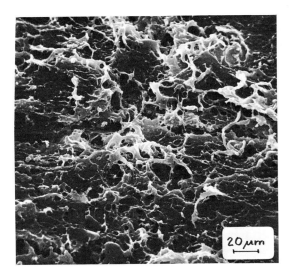

Fig. 7. Three week experiment. Increasing destruction of articular cartilage surface in the pressure center (×600)

In addition to the degenerative changes described, regenerative changes were now seen for the first time, namely the appearance of so-called atypical chondrones. Their appearance after variously caused degenerative changes in articular cartilage has been reported by sundry authors [1, 4] and has most often been regarded as evidence of inadequate regeneration of cartilage cells.

Increasing destructive changes were observed in the experiments lasting three and four weeks. Characteristic macroscopic surface changes now seen ranged from roughening to ulceration.

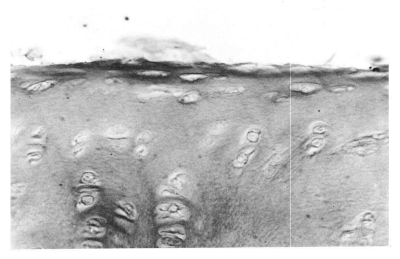

Fig. 8. Three week experiment. Ruptured tangential fiber layer with opened up lacunae, shrinking and necrosis of cells, and altered staining of ground substance (alcian blue PAS × 160)

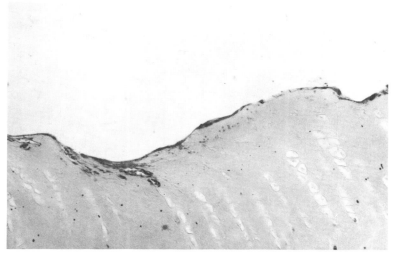

Fig. 9. Four week experiment. Arthrosis-like appearance (Goldner's stain × 63)

SEM of the articular surface now revealed increasing disintegration, with flaking of broad lamellae, tearing and fissuring, and rupturing and fragmentation of fibers. The latter no longer showed any orderly arrangement (Fig. 7). These changes in the articular cartilage surface are like those in arthrosis in man, seen in the scanning electron micrographs published by Cotta and Puhl, Ohnsorge, Schutz and Holm, McCall, and others. Similarly comparable are the histological appearance of fissuring and rupturing in the tangential zone, shrinking and necrosis of cells, and altered staining of ground substance (Figs. 8 and 9).

Because of the gradual transition from prearthrotic changes to arthrosis, precise morphological distinction between the two phases is impossible. However, the first microstructural damage observed, namely changes in the cell nuclei and an initial loss of ground substance which begins to expose bundles of collagen fibers, must be understood as the pathogenetic onset of a prearthrotic state.

As proved experimentally by various investigators [6, 10, 15, etc.] even just immobilization of a limb, with or without weight-bearing, itself causes degenerative changes in articular cartilage. The histological and scanning electron microscopic findings in the present investigations have confirmed this. Even in the two-week experiments, histological examination showed some changes in nuclear staining and slight shrinkage of chondrocytes in the tangential and intermediate zones, and SEM revealed circumscribed exposure of fibrillary structures. The typical surface contour pattern was preserved (Fig. 10).

The histological changes observed after four weeks were shrinking of cells, altered staining of ground substance in the tangential and intermediate zones, and rupturing of fibers in the tangential zone. SEM revealed obvious exposure of fibrillary structures, which showed rupturing and fragmentation, as well as surface flaking of lamellae (Fig. 11). These findings correspond to those seen in arthrosis.

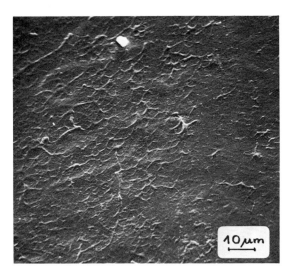

Fig. 10. Two week immobilization. Fiber structures are beginning to be exposed on the cartilage surface (× 1 000)

Although the results of experiments in animals cannot be directly applied to man, it does seem justifiable to assume that comparable degenerative changes in articular cartilage can be caused by therapeutic immobilization of the knee joint, e. g., in a walking plaster. This would correlate with clinical experience.

2. Distraction

Previous experimental studies of joint distraction in live subjects have produced two important conclusions. These are that distraction causes:
1. circumscribed local hyperemia
2. considerable intraarticular effusion with a variable blood content

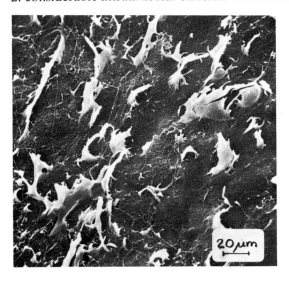

Fig. 11. Four week immobilization. Lamellar flaking of cartilage surface and rupturing of fibers (× 525)

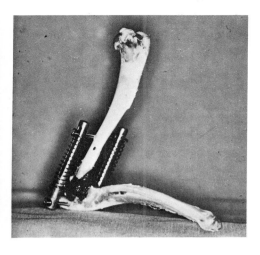

Fig. 12. Means of producing distraction of the elbow joint in the rabbit

The object of the present experiments was to study the effect in live animals of distracting joints with different degrees of force without greatly interfering with joint mobility.

Materials and Methods

Preliminary experiments showed the elbow joint of the rabbit to be particularly suitable. An apparatus was developed which produced distraction by measured spring force applied to both ends of Kirschner wires passing through the humerus and the olecranon. The joint capsule was not affected. The animals moved about without obvious difficulty (Fig. 12).

In the experiments performed on 154 fully grown animals, the distracting force in the first group was 0.35 Kp, corresponding to about one tenth of the animals body weight. In the second group it was 1.7 Kp, equivalant to about half the body weight. The duration of distraction varied from one week to eight weeks. The opposite elbow joint served as a control. At the end of each experiment the apparatus was removed and roentgenograms of both limbs were obtained. Angiographic, histological, vital staining, and SEM investigations were then completed.

Results and Discussion

1. The radiological investigations showed widening of the joint space in all cases. This widening was seen immediately after application of the distraction apparatus and it remained unchanged throughout each experiment. No changes in bone structure were detected. The distraction force of 1.7 Kp caused dislocation in some animals. These were excluded from further study.

2. Angiography using a Micropaque-Turnbull's blue mixture showed extensive dilatation of blood vessels, both arterial and venous, in the affected limb. This was confirmed radiologically and by stereomicroscopy using Spalteholz preparations. Extravasations, which might have been potential sources of the hemorrhages and hemorrhagic effusions yet to be described, were not found. The angiographic findings remained unchanged throughout the experiments and did not appear to depend on the distraction force used.

3. Hardly any histological change in hyaline cartilage was observed within four weeks. A rust-brown discoloration was seen macroscopically from the beginning of the second week and was associated with a loss of typical cartilage luster. This discoloration was attributed to the persisting hemarthrosis which developed immediately after the beginning of each experiment. Definite histological changes in cartilage were found only after eight weeks. These were in the tangential and intermediate zones. They included circumscribed surface defects, lacunae (some of which opened into the joint cavity), and hypochromasia of chondrocytes and amorphous ground substance. The intermediate zone showed collections of necrotic chondrocytes which looked a little like atypical chondrones (Fig. 13). The soft tissue changes helped to explain the cartilage changes. Thus hyperemia of the joint capsule and the periarticular muscles was present throughout the experiments. The joint capsule showed widespread diffuse or focal hemorrhages even after distraction applied for only a short period. These were followed by increasing synovitis and finally by capsular fibrosis. Histiocyte containing accumulations of hemosiderin were numerous. No vascular lesions were observed. Signs of atrophy seen in the subchondral cortical bone were another consequence of the joint distraction.

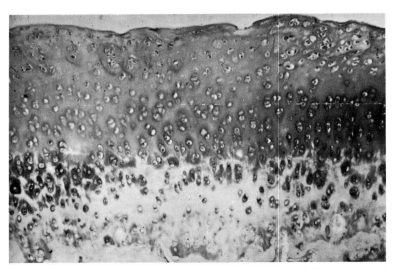

Fig. 13. Eight week distraction. Defects in the tangential fiber zone with opening up of lacunae. Altered staining of chondrocytes and cell nuclei. Pyknotic nuclei and shrinking of cells (astra blue-nuclear fast red × 100)

The findings in cartilage, bone, and soft tissue were dependent on the duration of action of the force, but not on its magnitude.

4. Vital staining of articular cartilage by methylene blue injected into the joint showed a slight reduction in the diffusion of the cationic dye during the entire period of distraction when the force used was 1.7 Kp. With a distraction force of 0.35 Kp an initial slight increase in diffusion rate was followed, in experiments lasting longer than two weeks, by a reduction in diffusion rate after that time.

5. SEM in the eight-week experiments revealed multiple areas of exposure of fibrillary structures. Their orderly arrangement was disturbed. However, there was no evidence of major disintegration of the articular surface.

From these findings, it can be concluded that the experimental distraction of joints by forces equal to about one tenth of the body weight (joint mobility being preserved) can cause structural changes, including changes in hyaline cartilage. These changes were related to the duration of the experiments. Understandably the changes in cartilage appeared only after prolonged joint distraction. Their genesis was probably multifactorial. Likely pathogenetic factors were capsular fibrosis, hemarthrosis, and diminished pressure and friction. Subsequent investigations have shown that all the changes caused by four weeks of distraction by a force of 0.35 Kp were completely reversible (8).

It thus appears that sudden widening of the joint space (which may also be a consequence of the clinical use of traction) was the decisive pathogenetic factor in the present experiments. However, clinical joint traction is not necessarily equally damaging. The clinical relevance of the experiments is naturally limited. Nevertheless, the findings could help to explain the known clinical effects of long-continued treatment by extension, namely periarticular edema, capsular swelling, joint effusion, local hyperemia, and bone atrophy.

Summary and Conclusions

In animal experiments, considerable pathologic changes in articular cartilage are caused by compression and immobilization and by distraction. As would be expected distraction causes less pronounced changes than compression and immobilization. It was shown that the extent of the changes was partly a function of the magnitude of the force used and was always a function of the duration of action of the force.

The microstructural changes in hyaline articular cartilage caused by compression and immobilization were most impressively demonstrated by scanning electron microscopy. First comes a loss of amorphous ground substance, with localized exposure of bundles of collagen fibrils. Next comes increasing disintegration of the cartilage surface until finally the appearance is comparable to that of arthrosis in man. The exposure of bundles of fibrils represents the first structural damage to the microarchitecture and as such it can be regarded as the pathogenetic beginning of a prearthrotic condition.

Depending on the duration of the experiment, immobilization alone (weight-bearing continuing) leads to degenerative changes in cartilage. This observation justifies a critical appraisal of the therapeutic immobilization of joints with continuing weight-bearing. As the investigations show, the structural pattern seen on the surface of healthy articular cartilage depends on a three-dimensional meshwork of collagen fibrils.

Joint distraction causes comparable degenerative changes in cartilage. These, however, are reversible within a limited period (four weeks).

It is evident from the changes produced by compression and immobilization and those produced by distraction, that, as Lindner affirms, hyaline articular cartilage reacts to different kinds of mechanical damage in a uniform manner.

References

1. Carlson, H.: Acta Orthop. Scand. Supplementum **28** (1957)
2. Clarke, J. C.: J. Anat. (Lond.) **108**, 23 (1971)
3. Cotta, H., Puhl, W.: Arch. orthop. Unfall-Chir. **68**, 152 (1970)
4. Crelin, E. S., Southwick, W. O.: Anat Rec. **149**, 113 (1964)
5. Dustmann, H. O., Puhl, W., Schulitz, K. P.: Arch. orthop. Unfall-Chir. **71**, 148 (1971)
6. Ely, L. W., Mensor, M. C.: Surg. Gynec. Obstet. **57**, 212 (1933)
7. Gardner, D. L., Woodward, D.: Ann rheum. Dis. **28**, 379 (1969)
8. Hackenbroch, M. H., Springer, H. H.: Z. Orthop. **112**, 140 (1974)
9. Lindner, J.: Verh. dtsch. orthop. Ges. **53**, 44 (1966)
10. Matthias, H. H., Glupe, J.: Arch. orthop. Unfall-Chir. **60**, 380 (1966)
11. McCall, J. G.: Lancet II 1968 II, 1194
12. Ohnsorge, J., Schütt, G., Holm, R.: Z. Orthop. **108**, 268 (1970)
13. Richter, J. E.: Beitr. elektronenmikroskop. Direkt-Abb. Oberfläche **2**, 575 (1971)
14. Salter, R. B., Field, P.: J. Bone Jt. Surg. **42 A**, 31 (1960)
15. Thaxter, T. H., Mann, R. A., Anderson, C. E.: J. Bone Jt. Surg. **47 A**, 3 (1965)
16. Titze, A.: Langenbecks Arch. Chir. **321**, 232 (1968)
17. Walcher, K., Stürz, H.: Arch. orthop. Unfall-Chir. **71**, 216 (1971)
18. Zarek, J. M., Edwards, J.: Med. Electron. Biol. Engng. **3**, 449 (1965)

Translation from the German: Die Reaktion des hyalinen Gelenkknorpels unter Druck, Immobilisation und Distraktion. In: Knorpelschaden am Knie, 4. Reisensburger Workshop zur klinischen Unfallchirurgie, edited by C. Burri and A. Rüter. In: Hefte zur Unfallheilkunde, Vol. 127 (1976). © Springer-Verlag 1976.

The Treatment of Acute Knee Ligament Injuries

G. Muhr, H. Tscherne, and L. Gotzen

The basic principle of treatment of acute knee ligament injuries is the restoration and preservation of joint stability. Ligament healing must be accompanied by careful attention to the surrounding muscles. In each case the importance of the injured structure, the degree of injury, and the measures necessary to obtain rapid healing must be taken into careful consideration.

Injuries may be divided into three stages: strains, sprains, and ruptures. If possible, long periods of immobilization should be avoided because of the danger of muscle atrophy. Approximately 84% of all injuries are strains or sprains [4]. Because of their frequency it is important to consider the optimal treatment of these less severe injuries.

Ligament Strains: These are managed by elastic bandages, analgesics, and antiinflammatory agents for 8–14 days. If an effusion is present with significant pain, the joint is aspirated and immobilized in a plaster slab. After 48–72 hours a walking cast is applied. This plaster should fit the contours of the leg well and its edges must be padded. The knee is flexed 10°–20°. Knees with previous injuries are immobilized for only 4–5 days to minimize the risk of muscle atrophy. Exercises are encouraged in plaster and continued after the plaster is removed. The patient should be observed for 2–3 weeks.

Sprains: Sprains with slight laxity can be difficult to differentiate from complete ruptures. There is a continuous transition from the sprain through an isolated rupture to complete capsular disruption. We feel that an angulation of 3° or more is an indication for surgery. *If less,* the management is essentially that of the simple strain.

Ligament Rupture: When stress X-ray shows significant instability, we favour surgical treatment for the following reasons:

1. Ligament injuries treated initially by surgery recover faster in our experience.

2. The accurate apposition of the torn ends reduces defective healing and thus improves the prognosis.

3. Surgery allows an accurate assessment of damage to neighboring structures such as menisci and articular cartilage.

4. Prompt diagnosis, suture, and early immobilization reduce the risk of further damage.

Surgical Technique

Ligament injuries should be repaired as early as possible. Rapid degeneration of the ligament ends makes delayed suture more difficult and even impossible after only two weeks. "Every day that elapses between accident and operation diminishes the success of the result"[6].

Bleeding should be controlled during surgery by meticulous hemostasis. Ligaments should be sutured by fine atraumatic material which is absorbable. Massive sutures do not improve stability and may interfere with blood supply. They may also cause granulomatous reactions.

When possible, ligaments should be reinserted into cancellous bone under a bony cortex (Fig. 1). Larger bony avulsions can simply be reattached with wires or screws. If the ligaments are shredded or weak, grafts or free transplants may be necessary.

Damage to other structures is treated at the same time. Detached but undamaged meniscii should be retained if possible and large fragments of cartilage reimplanted. In the case of fractures, restoration of the joint surfaces takes precedence over the ligament injury.

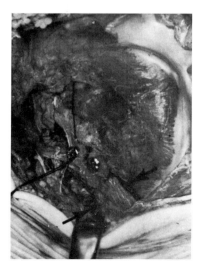

Fig. 1. Replacement of a periosteal avulsion of a collateral ligament underneath the cortex and reinforced with screws

Collateral Ligament Injuries

Simple collateral ligament injuries for the most part can be dealt with easily. They are best approached through longitudinal incisions. Superficial and deep portions of the ligament must be examined and the joint should be inspected at the same time. If adequate suture is impossible, then alternative methods must be considered (Fig. 2). Pedicle grafts, such as from the gracilis or biceps are

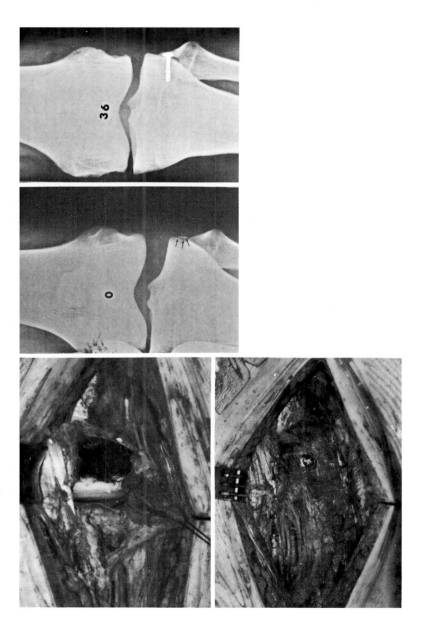

Fig. 2. Soccer injury with bony avulsion of the lateral capsular ligament apparatus. Avulsion of the anterior cruciate and medial meniscal lesion as well as damage to articular cartilage. Treatment consisted of reattaching the lateral avulsion with screws, reinsertion of the cruciate, and shaving of the cartilage. 36 weeks postoperatively the knee is stable

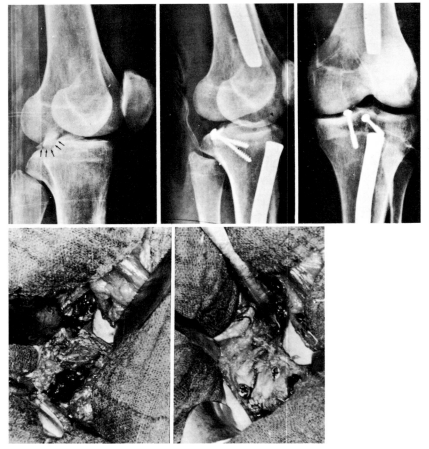

Fig. 3. Multiple injuries including right femoral and tibial fractures. Detachment of avulsed fragment from posterior cruciate ligament.

preferred over free grafts such as skin. The peroneal nerve should always be exposed in repairing lateral ligament lesions. It is especially important to attach capsular injuries to bone. This will prevent later rotational instability.

Cruciate Ligament Injuries

An isolated cruciate ligament injury is rare. If such a diagnosis is made, however, surgical treatment is indicated in practically every case. The only cruciate injury treated conservatively is an undisplaced bony avulsion with no instability.

The knee is opened through a parapatellar incision. In posterior cruciate injuries a popliteal incision may be necessary. Torn ligaments are reapposed by fine sutures and if accompanied by bony avulsions, they can be reinserted into drilled channels. Large fragments can be stabilized by means of screws (Figs. 3

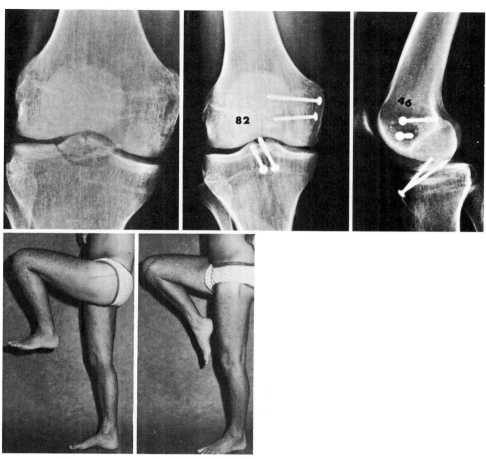

Fig. 4. Multiple injuries from motor vehicle accident including avulsion of medial collateral ligament and anterior tibial spine. Anatomic reconstruction with screws, normal function $1^1/_2$ years later

and 4). When repairing an anterior cruciate lesion the flexed knee should be held posteriorly; in treating a posterior cruciate ligament injury the knee must be pulled forward. If the cruciate ligament cannot be repaired we favor tunnel grafts from the patellar ligament as described by Bruckner, Jones [2, 5] or Augustine [1].

Multiple Ligament Injuries

Gross instability, which suggests combined ruptures, requires particularly careful attention. The exposure is through longitudinal parapatellar incisions. The branches of the saphenous nerve should be preserved if possible to prevent painful neuromas. Multiple ligament injuries are treated essentially as a series of individual lesions. Ruptures of all stabilizing structures produce major problems. In spite of careful technique the prognosis for such a massive injury is poor. Acute vascular damage is not uncommon or may appear a few days later as a thrombosis or a tear. An interarticular drain is used routinely after arthrotomy for 12–24 hours to avoid hemarthrosis. A plaster is usually applied with the knee at $140°-160°$.

Results

Between July 1st 1971 and December 31st 1975 62 patients with acute knee ligament injuries underwent surgical treatment. Of all the cases 22 were due to traffic accidents and 22 as a result of athletics. The average age was 36, ratio between men and women was 4:1. This shows that the ligament injury of the knee is a typical lesion of young adults and an optimal reconstruction is necessary. Of all the lesions 32 were isolated tears (15 medial, 6 lateral, 9 anterior cruciate lig., 2 post. cruc. lig.), 30 received multiple tears (16 anteromedial, 7 anterolateral, 2 posterolateral, 5 dislocations). In the 5 dislocations with complete instability, 3 cases were open and 2 were complicated by concomitant vessel lesions.

Operative treatment consisted of adapting ligament and capsule sutures, transosseous fixation of avulsed ligaments, and reattachment of osseous fragments by screws or wires. Also acute cartilage tears were adapted with atraumatic sutures.

In 2 open dislocations external fixation clamps were applied. Due to infection arthrodesis was necessary in one case, while the second healed with a slight functional loss but moderate instability. All other patients healed without complication.

55 of the 62 patients underwent a follow-up examination on average 26 months after accident. In isolated tears 27 our of the 28 patients controlled showed full stability and function.

In multiple ligament injuries only 18 out of the 27 patients showed excellent or good results. 6 cases with a significant loss of mobility were classified as moderate, 3 patients after complex instability or dislocation showed an unsatisfactory result because of pain, major instability or severe loss of function.

Altogether of the 55 patients with acute, simple and complex ligament injuries 72% showed excellent or good results, 13% were moderate and 5% poor.

A consistent therapeutic approach should be adopted to all cases of ligament injuries. Good results with surgical treatment can be achieved only through immediate intervention using good technique and atraumatic materials. A full postoperative regime is essential. Even in severe disruptions such as dislocations the results of surgery are far superior to the results of conservative or later reconstructive measures (Fig. 5).

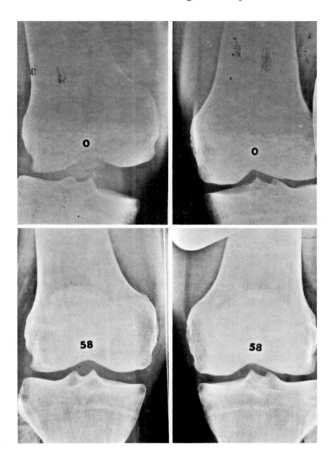

Fig. 5. Tibial ligament injury, medial ligament complex and both cruciates sustained playing soccer. Ligament repair and reinsertion of cruciates. Stable knee one year later

References

1. Augustine, R. W.: The Unstable Knee. Amer. J. Surg. **92**, 380 (1956).
2. Brückner, H.: Eine neue Methode der Kreuzbandplastik. Chirurg **37**, 413 (1966).
3. Burri, C., Helbing, G., Rüter, A.: Die Behandlung der posttraumatischen Bandinstabilität am Kniegelenk. Orthopäde **3**, 184 (1974).
4. Jonasch, E.: Das Kniegelenk. Berlin: Walter de Gruyter 1964.
5. Jones, K.-G.: Reconstruction of The Anterior Cruciate Ligament. J. Bone Jt. Surg. **45 A**, 925 (1963).
6. O'Donoghue, D. H.: Treatment of Injuries to Athletes. Philadelphia-London-Toronto: Saunders 1970.
7. Tscherne, J., Szyszkowitz, R.: Verletzungen der Gelenke und paraartikulären Gewebe. In: Chirurgie der Gegenwart. München–Berlin–Wien: Urban und Schwarzenberg 1974.

Updated Translation from the German: Therapie frischer Bandverletzungen. In: Bandverletzungen am Knie, 3. Reisensburger Workshop zur klinischen Unfallchirurgie, edited by C. Burri and A. Rüter. In: Hefte zur Unfallheilkunde, Vol. 125 (1975). © Springer-Verlag 1975.

The Rehabilitation of Knee Ligament Injuries

C. Burri, G. Helbing, and W. Spier

For years Böhler and his school advocated a purely conservative treatment of acute knee ligament injuries. They still favor this approach to many injuries. Immobilization in plaster was the mainstay of treatment. The period of immobilization was determined by the degree of instability and could be up to sixteen weeks in duration. The knee was immobilized in $10° - 15°$ of flexion. Böhler and Jonasch [5] claim that even long periods of immobilization do not result in quadriceps atrophy, providing that the patient walked with the cast and performed isometric exercises. We could not confirm either the position of immobilization or the lack of quadriceps atrophy. It is our opinion that a systematic active exercise treatment is important to overcome stiffness and to strengthen the quadriceps, particularly after a period of immobilization.

Böhler [1] recommends the knee-bending frame that he has developed. The height of the padded crosspiece is adjusted so that the heel no longer touches the base. A sling is attached above the ankle joint and tied to a handle. The patient can then let the knee hang until he feels pain. This allows both active and passive stretching of the joint. The majority of the action, however, is performed by gravity.

A similar principle of combined active passive motion is the "Frankfurt – motion splint." Again the patient often exercises mainly his arm and avoids bending his knee by lifting the pelvis. Once the knee is mobile, gymnastics, stairs, and the stationary bicycle become advisable forms of exercise.

Böhler has stated that no exercise must cause pain. Passive movement, massage, and excessive heat must be avoided if they produce pain and secondary chronic irritation. Cold is used more and more frequently in the stiff knee. Pool therapy including gymnastics and swimming are especially helpful.

O'Donoghue [7] and many others suggest that in acute knee ligament injuries surgery has definite advantages. Surgery is also followed by 4–12 weeks of immobilization and certainly the difficulties of immobilization are not lessened by the ligament suture.

Effects of Immobilization

Immobilization of the knee has serious disadvantages for the muscles of the thigh and leg, especially the quadriceps atrophy. Not only is the leg weaker but the loss of muscle tone hinders the stability of the knee joint. The fact that muscles can stabilize joints is demonstrated by American football players that continue to play in spite of absent cruciate ligaments. Moreover the musculature protects freshly sutured or healed ligaments from overstrain and should, therefore, be encouraged to function in the early stages after ligaments suture.

Immobilization leads to considerable impairment in the knee mobility. The rehabilitation of such a stiffened knee is often a lengthy process taxing the perseverance and patience of the patient.

The ligaments themselves are weakened by lack of knee function. Laros and his coworkers [6] showed a significant loss of strength in the knee ligaments of dogs after immobilization for as little as six weeks. The cause was subperiosteal bone resorption at the points of origin and insertion of the ligaments. On the other hand, training increased the thickness of the ligaments and the number of collagen fibers.

Articular cartilage does not survive immobilization without damage. Hall (4) found degenerative changes at the contact surfaces, while connective tissue membranes formed on the cartilage zones which were not utilized or in contact.

Dustmann and Puhl [3] showed that hemarthrosis damaged cartilage. The injection of an animal's own blood produced definite electron microscope changes of roughness of articular surfaces, fragmentation of collagen fibers, and loss of cross striations. Immobilization of the joint increased the degenerative changes. Destruction is presumably caused by enzymes in the hemarthrosis and has been interpreted as a prearthrois. This suggests that early aspiration and mobilization are the treatment methods of choice.

Effects of Early Mobilization

The preservation of joint function following meticulous reduction of fractures and early movement has been known for some time. It was, therefore, obvious to search for a way to allow early motion soon after ligament surgery. Obviously free and unrestrained motion of the knee joint after ligament suture or reconstruction is not feasible, as the suture line would be overstrained. It was, therefore, decided to test experimentally whether a restricted range of motion could be allowed without endangering either ligament repair or reconstruction. During ligament repair, it was noted that the ligaments were only tight when in full extension or the extreme of flexion, but they were rather lax during intermittent stages. It was decided initially to determine the range of movement which allowed the sutured ligaments to remain relatively lax.

Experimental Findings

In human amputation and cadaver preparations the individual ligaments of the knee were severed and then joined with fine rubber sutures. The range of motion was measured which would barely put tension upon this suture line. The lateral ligaments were divided·at their midpoint while the cruciates were dissected out at their distal point of origin. This showed that various ligaments became taut at very different degrees of movement of the knee joint. The lateral collateral ligament permitted the widest range of motion while the tibial collateral ligament allowed the least. The study revealed that no tension was present on any of the four knee ligaments between 20°–60° of flexion, but every varus or valgus motion, rotation or drawer movement endangered the suture line.

In a second experiment the tibial collateral and anterior cruciate ligaments of three freshly amputated legs were severed. These ligaments had shown the least tolerance to flexion and are also the most frequently injured. The ligaments were then sutured and under controlled humidity they were moved 430,000 times between a range of 20°–60° of flexion. This is equivalant to a 200 Km walk. The suture line in all three preparations remained undamaged.

Finally a third experiment was carried out on animals. The medial collateral ligament of the knee of ten rabbits was sectioned through two-thirds of its width. Five of the animals were allowed to move freely and the other five were placed in a circular plaster for three weeks. At the end of three weeks the medial collateral ligament of both groups were healed. There was no instability of the joint. The histological picture of the fibroblasts in continuous motion showed an orderly formation. In absolute immobilization, however, the fibroblasts presented an uneven picture (Fig. 1 a and b).

These experiments suggest that active mobility is desirable immediately after knee joint surgery, either acute ligament repair or ligament reconstruction. It suggests that movement itself neither endangers the suture line nor delays healing. Care must be taken to prevent the last 20° of extension and to not allow flexion past 60°. Valgus and varus movement, rotation, and drawering must also be totally restricted.

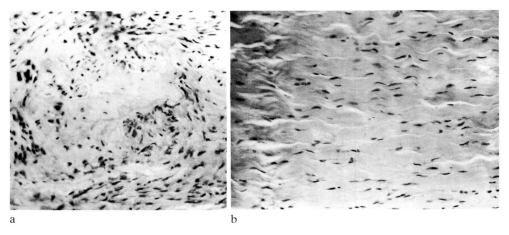

a   b

Fig. 1. Medial collateral of rabbit 3 weeks after division. (a) Uneven scar formation during immobilization in plaster as shown in histologic preparation; (b) functional treatment shows resulting lengthwise scar formation

Technique of Early Mobilization

We have constructed a plaster cast which permits limited mobility [2]. Initially a circular plaster from thigh to toes is applied in the usual manner. A cylinder is then removed leaving approximately 15 cm of the knee exposed. With the aid of a sighting mechanism hinges are now fitted on both sides which have stops to limit extension to 20° and flexion to 60° (Fig. 2). The rotational axis lies at the level of the femoral condyle, i.e., approximately $1\frac{1}{2}$ cm above the joint line. After these hinges have been fastened with plaster bandages and are secure, the cast permits walking and the patients are allowed to move and bear weight within the prescribed range. The clinical results after ligament repairs treated with such a limited motion cast are encouraging.

Our present program for the rehabilitation of ligament repairs or reconstructions is as follows: Immediately postoperatively a compression bandage is applied to the limb, the limb is placed in a posterior splint in 20° of flexion. This splint is removed twice daily by the surgeon and the patient makes gentle flexion which may not exceed 60°. Drains are removed after 24 h and any effusion is cautiously aspirated. Seven to ten days following surgery, the limited motion cast is applied, and the patient wears it for an average of five weeks (Fig. 3). Following removal of the limited motion cast, only a short period of active exercises is needed until the knee can be bent beyond the right angle and fully extended. Atrophy has been avoided and the sutured ligaments are stable and capable of bearing stress.

Until full mobility is obtained the usual conservative measures are adopted. Swimming and motion exercises in water are especially valuable.

Recently the use of a light cast has considerably simplified the application and wearing of a limited motion cast. This synthetic material which hardens under ultraviolet radiation has only half the weight of plaster but is much harder. In

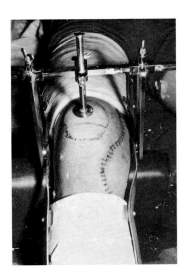

Fig. 2. Application of limited-motion cast. *1*. Walking cast on thigh. *2*. Cutting out cylinder above knee. *3*. Fitting of joint splints with sighting mechanism

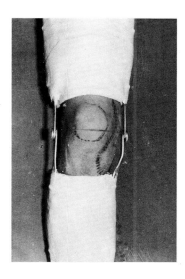

Fig. 3. The limited-motion cast permits a swing between 20° and 60° flexion and is used as a cast permitting walking

our experience the weak points of a limited motion cast are the ankle and the fixation of the hinges. Light casts allow more firm fixation of the metal hinges. Even motion in water and swimming are possible. The cast must be dried by hot air so that the moist padding material does not macerate the skin. The removal of a light cast with an oscillating saw causes no problems. The hinges can be removed and used again. The only caution advised in using the light cast material is the possibility of pressure points and therefore careful padding is required.

Summary

Today the general feeling is that complete ligament reconstruction combined with careful rehabilitation offers the best results with both acute and late ligament reconstructions. Prolonged immobilization after surgery has definite disadvantages. Cadaver and animal experimentations show that ligament sutures and reconstructions experience no stress at the suture line if the range of motion is kept between 20° and 60° and if varus, valgus, rotation, and drawer movements are avoided.

On the basis of these facts we have constructed a limited motion cast which permits a range of motion between 20° and 60° and eliminated the other dangers. To date this device has yielded good results in over 100 patients.

References

1. Böhler, L.: Technik der Knochenbruchbehandlung, 3. Band. Wien: Maudrich 1944
2. Burri, C., Pässler, H. H., Radde, J.: Experimentelle Grundlagen zur funktionellen Behandlung nach Bandnaht und -plastik am Kniegelenk. Z. Orthop. **111,** 378 (1973)

3. Dustmann, H. O., Puhl, W.: Haemarthros und Arthrose. Langenbecks Arch. Chir. Suppl. **111,** 47 (1971)
4. Hall, M. C.: Cartilage Changes after Experimental Immobilization of the Knee Joint of the Young Patient. J. Bone. Jt. Surg. **45 A,** 36 (1963)
5. Jonasch, E.: Das Kniegelenk. Berlin: de Gruyter 1964
6. Laros, G. S., Tipton, C. M., Cooper, R. R.: Influence of Physical Activity on Ligament Insertions in the Knee of Dogs. J. Bone Jt. Surg. **53 A,** 275 (1971)
7. O'Donoghue, D. H.: The Unhappy Triad. Amer. J. Orthop. **6,** 242 (1964)

Translation from the German: Nachbehandlung nach Kniebandverletzungen. In: Bandverletzungen am Knie, 3. Reisensburger Workshop zur klinischen Unfallchirurgie, edited by C. Burri and A. Rüter. In: Hefte zur Unfallheilkunde, Vol. 125 (1975). © Springer-Verlag 1975.

Rotational Stability of the Knee

W. Müller

Introduction

The assessment of an unstable knee and of the resulting handicap is governed by the demands made on the knee by the individual's activities.

In his textbook "Die funktionelle Behandlung der Knochenbrüche und Gelenkverletzungen" ("The functional treatment of fractures and joint injuries") (1919), Steinmann gave only two pages to ruptures of the medial ligament of the knee. Under this heading he wrote as follows: "If I devote a few words to the diagnosis of such a common injury, this is due to the fact that the diagnosis is frequently unrecognized and that it has some bearing on treatment. The injury is in fact very often mistaken for a cartilage lesion and is often operated upon under that diagnosis. Ruptures of the medial ligament of the knee must be treated conservatively. Various surgeons have made attempts at operative treatment designed to bring the ends of the ligament together, but such procedures are not worthwhile because the rupture is usually not complete and if the mobilization treatment which I recommend is carried out the medial ligament will regain its normal strength."

He goes on to give four examples illustrating how these ligamentous injuries were treated. Compression bandages were applied for about two weeks, after which active movements were cautiously resumed and massage was started. Nowadays, in view of the importance attached to fitness for sport and the general demand for full restoration of functional capacity, these opinions are no longer acceptable.

Steinmann claimed good results from his method of treatment, better at least than those achieved in many patients whose knees were immobilized in plaster for long periods. He asserted that persistent slackness of the medial ligament with an abnormal range of abduction at the knee joint was seen only in cases of complete rupture or surgical division of the ligament distant from its insertion. In such cases he claimed to have restored the function of the medial ligament by means of a pedicled osteoperiosteal graft from the medial side of the tibia.

In 1951 the situation was still fundamentally the same. In his writings on orthopaedic surgery Lange simply remarks that when dealing with an unstable knee the surgeon must note whether the laxity is on the medial or the lateral side, so that he can direct his treatment appropriately.

If we were content to tackle the problem using such methods the results would certainly not come up to modern expectations. It is to the credit of workers, such as Smillie [32, 33], O'Donoghue [20–22], Helfet [8], Ficat [5, 6], and others, that a systematic study of the injuries of the ligamentous capsule of the knee was at last undertaken.

When he introduced his concept of the "unhappy triad", O'Donoghue [22] showed that the patterns of injury invariably have complex causal interrelationships. Today we know that an unhappy triad is not always an unhappy triad, but that the lesions, although interrelated, are much more varied than is implied by the combination of anterior cruciate ligament + medial ligament + meniscus. It must be emphasized that the meniscus lesion, as O'Donoghue described it, is seldom a lesion of the avascular cartilaginous meniscus alone, but in most cases involves a tear of the attachment of the meniscus to the joint capsule. (Ligamentum collaterale posterius, described by H. Meyer, 1853). This type of "cartilage lesion" must be treated by suturing, because the injury is situated in the vascular region of the ligament in the joint capsule and healing is, therefore, possible. Trillat [34–37] subsequently demonstrated that the "pentade malheureuse" may also occur as a later development of these complex lesions.

New insights of this kind provided a foundation for further progress and it has now become possible to differentiate with greater precision between the various forms of instability which may persist as late sequelae after such injuries.

It is probably no coincidence that much of this work has been carried out in the USA and in France. One factor common to both countries is their enthusiasm for professional football — American football and rugby respectively. These sports produce unusually large numbers of complex knee injuries because in certain situations the rules of the game permit a player to neutralize an opponent by the "cross body block", often against the extended knee joint. These athletes want complete restitution of function after such accidents and expect their knees to be stable so that they can play without pain.

O'Donoghue [20–22], Slocum [30, 31], Hughston [11–13], Nicholas [18, 19], and Kennedy in the USA and Canada, and Trillat, Dejour, and Bousquet [36] in France have published valuable contributions on the rotational stability of the knee. At a very early stage in their work they obviously recognized that the simple and oldfashioned classification into adduction or abduction laxity, or anterior and posterior drawer signs was no longer sufficient to explain the persisting symptoms and functional incapacity which often follow such complex injuries.

Physiology and Pathophysiology

The Inevitable Sequence of Rotational Movements in the Knee

All extension or flexion movements of the knee joint are inevitably accompanied by rotational movements, depending on the position of the knee. Between the two extreme positions, flexion-valgus-external rotation and flexion-varus-internal rotation, there is a wide range in which all intermediate positions are feasible without overstraining the ligamentous capsule (Fig. 1). In the fully extended position all such movements are totally suspended, because the joint is locked by the internal rotation of the femur on the tibia which takes place as automatic terminal rotation in the last degrees of extension.

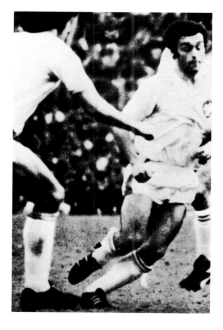

Fig. 1. Varus-flexion-internal rotation and valgus-flexion-external rotation at the knee joints illustrated in a footballer. The left leg, carrying the weight of the body, is in varus-flexion-internal rotation, while the right leg, with which he is about to kick the ball, is in valgus-flexion-external rotation

Passive Elements of Rotational Stability

There is no single anatomic element of the knee which is solely responsible for rotational stability. On the contrary, we must visualize the entire saucer, consisting of the head of the tibia, the menisci, the capsular apparatus, the fat pads, the patella, and the cruciate ligaments as an extended socket in which the condyles can rotate within fixed limits (Fig. 2). We must also assume that the cruciate ligaments serve as a hinge point for these movements and that they stabilize the axis of rotation too (Fig. 3).

The axis of rotation shifts even in the normal knee and cannot be localized within narrow limits. It is almost impossible to specify where the usual position

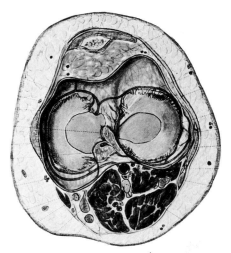

Fig. 2. The lower surface of the knee joint is really a saucer. Its base is formed by the tibia, while the menisci, the capsule, the fat pads, and the various tendons serve as soft tissue extensions at its edges

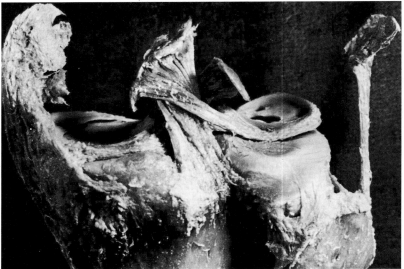

Fig. 3. The collateral and cruciate ligaments. In this illustration the latter have the appearance of fans

of the rotational axis is situated in ordinary movements, and it is still more difficult to determine where this axis may lie under extreme conditions. For this reason the literature contains widely varying statements regarding the site of the rotational axis.

The menisci constitute another very important element for the containment and braking of these rotatory movements in the tibial saucer (Fig. 4). The more one knows about the knee, the more one realizes that the menisci cannot be regarded as functioning in isolation. When deciding whether an operation is necessary, it is quite wrong for the surgeon to think solely in terms of the menisci and their removal. He must always bear in mind that they are a part of the extraordinarily complex stabilizing mechanism of the knee joint.

Every meniscectomy carries a risk of increased rotational instability on the side of the meniscus which has been removed.

After the menisci, the next components which we must consider are the fat pads. As soon as the quadriceps contracts and the tension in its tendon begins to rise, there is automatically an increase in the internal pressure in the fat pad

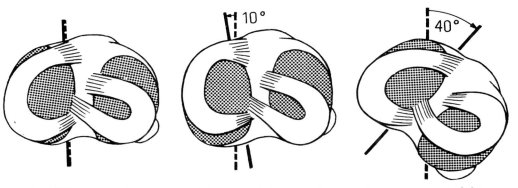

Fig. 4. The range of movement of the menisci during various rotatory movements of the femur on the tibia. Various end-positions are depicted

itself. From this instant onward it is no longer merely a soft and mechanically inert space-filler, but, consolidated by the rise in internal pressure, it assumes a braking function. Under conditions of maximal stress it acts as a shock absorber which damps out peak loads and brakes extreme movements.

The basin formed by the two semilunar cartilages and the fat pad is enclosed by a joint capsule of exceedingly complex structure, which incorporates an extraordinarily varied and beautifully designed network of fibers. If we analyse the directions in which these fibers run, again and again we find them arranged in the form of V-shaped triangular structures (Fig. 5).

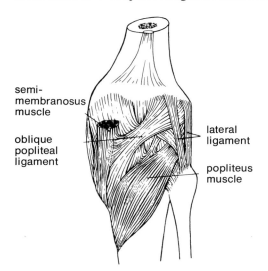

semi-
membranosus
muscle

oblique
popliteal
ligament

lateral
ligament

popliteus
muscle

Fig. 5. Number of the anatomic structures in the posterior capsule of the joint arranged in the form of a V. The collateral ligament itself may be V-shaped and, more important, the reflected portion of the semimembranosus tendon extends as a V-shaped radiation into the oblique popliteal ligament. Even the radiating strands of the popliteus tendon are arranged in a V-shaped pattern

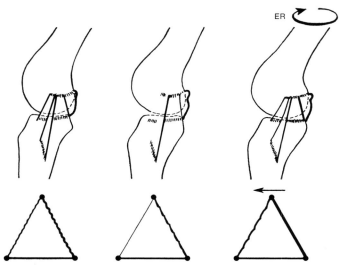

Fig. 6. The strength of a triangular structure with the modes of tension associated with rotation in various directions (ER = external rotation)

Owing to these fiber systems it is possible, as will be seen from the diagram, for the capsule itself to maintain a considerable degree of rotational stabilization (Fig. 6). It is, therefore, easy to understand how even the slightest stretching or residual laxity of the joint capsule will result in an increased range of potential rotation in the individual divisions of the joint, quite apart from any slight lateral instability which it may allow.

Active Element of Rotational Movement and Rotational Stabilization

The Quadriceps Extensor Apparatus, the Patella, and the Patellar Tendon

The physiological valgus of the extensor apparatus is responsible for the fact that every contraction of this powerful muscle exerts a rotational influence on the knee joint (Fig. 7). In the standing position with some degree of flexion, as the tibia is fixed, the patella pushes the lateral femoral condyle backward and thus causes external rotation of the femur. Alternatively, if the leg is free, the tibia is internally rotated on the femur. This mechanism is independent of the automatic terminal rotation at complete extension.

All well-trained athletes have an extremely well-developed vastus medialis and quadriceps with which they can exert active control over this special rotatory action of the patella and patellar ligament *whatever the angle of flexion* of the knee joint (Fig. 8).

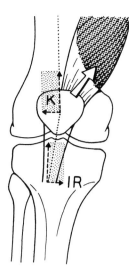

Fig. 7. Diagram showing the valgus arrangement of the quadriceps tendon with its rotatory effect on the distal end of the femur when the leg is fixed, a mechanism which in flexion is independent of automatic terminal rotation (K = force; IR = internal rotation)

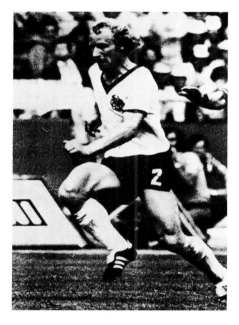

Fig. 8. This illustration shows how the vastus medialis is fully active even when the knee is flexed to approximately 110°

Pes Anserinus Muscle Group

The tendon insertion of this triple group of muscles is situated on the medial side, separated by a definite interval from the patellar ligament. The sartorius, the gracilis, and the semitendinosus exert an active effect on rotation. In the extended position their leverage makes only a small contribution toward rotation, but with increasing flexion it becomes stronger. In the same degree as their rotatory potential increases with flexion of the knee, their lateral stabilizing

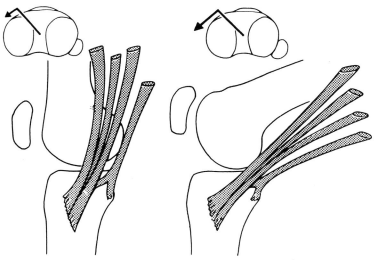

Fig. 9. How the rotatory action of the pes anserinus muscle group alters during extension and flexion. As flexion increases, its leverage becomes greater and its rotatory action more powerful

effect decreases. In the position of extension they come to lie almost parallel to the collateral ligament (Fig. 9).

Semimembranosus Tendon

This muscle is inserted into the medial condyle of the tibia at a point posterior and somewhat proximal to the insertion of the pes anserinus group. It too is an important internal rotator of the tibia. In addition, it has a reflected portion which radiates directly into the posterior capsule of the knee joint and the oblique popliteal ligament, so that it has the effect of tightening the capsule especially during flexion. This is still another V-shaped component which is built into the posterior capsule to ensure rotational stabilization.

The Iliotibial Tract

On the lateral side of the knee this is the most important structure concerned in anterior and lateral stabilization apart from the patellar ligament. The tract can be fully tightened by the action of the quadriceps and the hip muscles. Its importance in lateral and anterolateral stability of the knee must not be underestimated.

Biceps Femoris

The insertion of the biceps tendon into the head of the fibula lies further laterally. Like the muscles of the pes anserinus group, it provides lateral

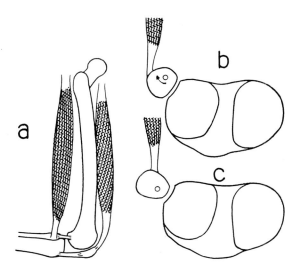

Fig. 10. Dislocation of the head of the fibula, a condition which may occur from the rotatory action of the biceps tendon when the knee joint is fully flexed

stabilization in extension and has a significant rotatory action in flexion. Because of its long leverage, it is an extremely powerful external rotator of the tibia when the knee is flexed to 90°. Occasionally this vigorous rotatory action, besides causing external rotation of the tibia on the femur, may cause external rotation of the head of the fibula on the tibia; a movement which may result in dislocation of the head of the fibula (Fig. 10).

Popliteus Muscle

This very powerful tendon, which arises deep to the lateral ligament on the lateral condyle of the femur, can pull the condyle externally and backward, thus making an important contribution to rotational stabilization. With the leg hanging free, the muscle acts as an internal rotator of the tibia on the femur. When the foot is fixed, the popliteus acts as a stabilizer of the lateral part of the knee joint by causing external rotation of the femur on the tibial plateau. Viewed from the side, the tendon then runs practically parallel to the posterior cruciate ligament and prevents drawer movements. In addition to its main tendon which arises from the condyle, the popliteus muscle possesses two other important tendinous strands, one of which pulls the lateral meniscus backward while the other is a powerful tightener of the posterior capsule.

Nicholas [18, 19] has classified the active and passive components concerned in medial and lateral stabilization into two "quadruple complexes."

The medial quadruple complex consists of:
– the medial ligament,
– the pes anserinus comprising sartorius, gracilis,
  and semitendinosus,
– the semimembranosus and
– the medial part of the posterior capsule with the oblique ligament.

The lateral quadruple complex consists of:
– the iliotibial tract,
– the popliteal muscle,
– the biceps femoris muscle and
– the fibular collateral ligament (lateral ligament).

The fact that these structures actually participate in the stabilization of the knee joint in various positions of rotation can be made perfectly clear by watching footballers engaged in various maneuvers with their limbs in special rotation conditions. It is apparent that the rotators come into action even during extension movements performed to control or pass the ball. Although they are, as flexors, antagonists of the quadriceps, their muscle bellies contract powerfully to produce the required rotation. On the medial side this applies to the pes anserinus group and the semimembranosus, and on the lateral side to the iliotibial tract and the biceps, which is often extremely prominent.

Varieties of Instability: Simple and Complex

The term simple instability denotes abnormal and excessive mobility about one axis only. Most such patients have a moderate degree of abduction and adduction laxity. The violence applied to the knee has caused a tear but has stopped short of completely rupturing the joint capsule. In these cases there is a place for conservative therapy, generally along functional lines.

In cases of complex instability, on the other hand, the joint can be put through an abnormal range of movement about several different axes. For example, there may be abduction laxity when the knee is fully extended; when flexed it can be opened with a snap. Furthermore the drawer sign is positive, often both forward and backward.

The drawer sign provides a means of diagnosing rotational instability. All surgeons are familiar with the clear-cut anterior and posterior drawer signs and must now elicit these by Slocum's technique with the knee in various positions of rotation. The examiner sits on the patient's foot to fix it in the chosen position – internal rotation, the neutral position or external rotation (not extreme internal or external rotation). With the leg in these positions he then elicits the drawer sign, both anteriorly and posteriorly (Fig. 11).

In this way it is generally possible to demonstrate excessive movement of the tibia on the condyles in one direction or another. These forms of rotational instability can be divided into four categories:
1. anteromedial rotational instability
2. anterolateral rotational instability
3. posterolateral rotational instability
4. posteromedial rotational instability

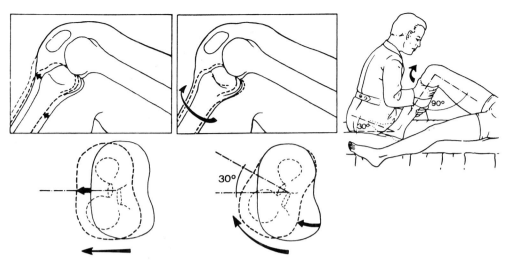

Fig. 11. The difference between a true anterior drawer sign and a rotational drawer sign

Their relative frequency is in the order listed above, i.e., anteromedial rotational instability is the commonest and posteromedial the rarest.

One theoretical point of particular interest is the behavior of the axis of rotation in these abnormalities. In such patients it is extremely difficult to locate the axis of rotation with precision, and it tends to shift from the unstable compartment of the knee toward the more stable side. For example, in anteromedial instability it moves forward and laterally, in anterolateral instability it moves forward and medially, and in the posterior forms of rotational instability it is displaced backward and either medially or laterally.

Surgical Methods of Reconstruction

To the best of my knowledge, Slocum in his publication on anteromedial rotatory instability was the first to advocate a specific operation to stabilize these rotational drawer movements. In his operation he rotates the pes anserinus tendon group proximally in such a way that the flexors are converted predominantly into internal rotators. Their active contraction is intended to overcome the passive instability. A new idea, that of active tendon transplantation, was thus developed into a clear and comprehensive technical procedure. Active tendon transplantation is based on the fact that active compensation of an unstable knee can be achieved by muscles and tendons, e.g., the quadriceps. In active tendon transplantation surgery the muscles used to stabilize the joint (e.g., muscles from the medial or lateral quadruple complexes) are attached to a new point of insertion which gives them better leverage for their new function.

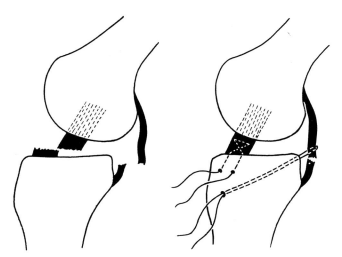

Fig. 12. This diagram shows the importance of the posterior capsule and the anterior cruciate ligament in maintaining forward stability

Trillat [34–37] claims good results from the operation devised by Slocum [31] in conjunction with medialization of the tibial tubercle by Elmslie's technique. However, when these forms of anteromedial rotatory instability are combined with undue valgus laxity, this method of stabilization is no longer adequate and a more elaborate operation of the kind described by O'Donoghue [20–22] is required. In such operations the entire medial and posterior capsule must be detached from the tibia and fixed to a new attachment further distally. As compared with reconstructive operations on single ligaments this procedure has the advantage that the entire capsular complex with its elaborate fiber structures is shifted distally and the surgeon is not restricted merely to reconstructing a single ligament (Fig. 12).

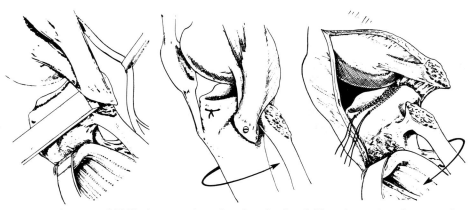

Fig. 13. Diagram of Trillat's operation, showing the feasibility of securing the posterior capsule

For the lateral side, where *anterolateral* instability is combined with laxity in the varus direction, I have found that Trillat's procedure is valuable (Fig. 13). In this operation a sagittal cut is made through the head of the fibula in such a way that the joint-bearing portion on the tibial side remains attached to the shaft of the fibula, while a bone fragment carrying the insertion of the lateral collateral ligament and the biceps tendon is detached and reimplanted at a new point further distally and further forward on the tibia, where it is secured with screws. In cases where the factors on the lateral side governing the instability are very complex, it may be advisable to work backward on this side, detaching the capsule and ligaments from the tibia and reinserting them further distally.

Conclusions

It is hardly necessary to say that the choice between the various operative procedures demands the utmost familiarity with methods of examination and surgical techniques. In arriving at a diagnosis, the surgeon must assess every component of the joint.

What is the condition of the menisci? In the ideal case the operation for transposition of the joint capsule to a line further distally along the tibia can be completed without difficulty only when a meniscectomy has previously been performed because of the injury or if the meniscus has to be removed during the operation because it is torn. In a few cases it may be possible to separate the meniscus together with the internal layer of the capsule by blunt dissection to such an extent that the external layers of the capsule together with the intermediate and long fiber strands can be reimplanted further distally.

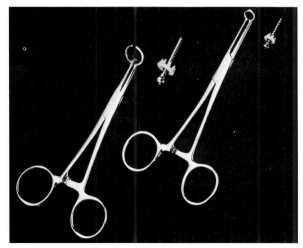

Fig. 14. The spiked ring or washer used with a screw for fixing avulsed ligaments or reimplanting ligaments detached with a thin layer of bone

During the last few years I have developed a system for reinforcing detached capsular and ligamentous structures. This is based on a special washer which has been made to fit the AO screws which I use. At the periphery of this washer is a ring of spikes with which the soft parts can be firmly held and securely fastened to the bone (Fig. 14). There is in principle no difference between the repair of a recent injury, where the torn tissues are in a state suitable for this mode of fixation, and an elective operation where the capsule has been deliberately detached with this fixation technique in mind.

As I have recently adopted the practice of detaching a thin layer of bone together with the capsule, it is often possible, once the bone has been secured in its new position, to manage the patient postoperatively without immobilization in plaster. This represents a further advance toward genuine functional treatment of these grave post-traumatic conditions of the knee joint. In all reconstructive procedures the best results are achieved when the lesions are systematically explored and the anatomic structures are reinstated as closely as possible to normal.

References

1. Bandi, W.: Helv. chir. acta Suppl. **11** (1972)
2. Burri, C., Hutschenreuter, P., Radde, J.: Excerpta med. **298,** 4 (1973)
3. Castaing, J., Burdin, Ph., Mougin, M.: Rev. Chir. orthop. **58,** Suppl. (1972)
4. Debeyre, J., Artigou, J. M.: Rev. Chir. orthop. **59,** 641 (1973)
5. Ficat, P.: Pathologie Fémoro-Patellaire. Paris: Masson 1970
6. Ficat, P.: Pathologie des Ménisques et des Ligaments du Genou. Paris: Masson 1962)
7. Goodfellow, J. W., Hungerford, D., Woods, G. C., Zindel, M: J. Bone Jt. Surg. **56 B,** 198 (1974)
8. Helfet, A. J.: The Management of Internal Derangement of the Knee. Philadelphia: Lippincott 1963
9. Henche, H. R.: Z. Orthop. **111,** 523 (1973)
10. Höhndorf: Med. Sport **12,** Heft 3 (1972)
11. Hughston, J. C.: J. Bone Jt. Surg. **50 B,** 1003 (1968)
12. Hughston, J. C., Eilers, A. F.: J. Bone Jt. Surg. **55 A,** 923 (1973)
13. Hughston, J. C., Stone, M., Andrews, J. R.: J. Bone Jt. Surg. **55 A,** 1318 (1973)
14. Ingwersen, O. S. (Ed.): The Knee Joint. Amsterdam: Excerpta Medica 1974. New York: American Elsener Publishing
15. Jani, L., Müller, W., Dolanc, B.: Ther. Umsch. **30,** 260 (1972)
16. Morscher, E., Müller, W.: Ther. Umsch. **31,** 227 (1974)
17. Müller, W.: Das Kniegelenk des Fußballers. Orthopäde **3,** 193 (1974)
18. Nicholas, J. A., Freiberger, R. H., Killoran, P. J.: J. Amer. med. Ass. **212,** 2236 (1970)
19. Nicholas, J. A.: J. Bone Jt. Surg. **55 A,** 899 (1973)
20. O'Donoghue, D. H.: J. Bone Jt. Surg. **32 A,** 721 (1950)
21. O'Donoghue, D. H.: J. Bone Jt. Surg. **48 A,** 503 (1966)
22. O'Donoghue, D. H.: J. Bone Jt. Surg. **55 A,** 941 (1973)
23. Ogden, J. A., Southwick, W. O.: J. Bone Jt. Surg. **55 A,** 1319 (1973)
24. Owen, R.: J. Bone Jt. Surg. **50 B,** 342 (1968)
25. Pipkin, G.: Clin. Orthop. **74,** 161 (1971)
26. Pipkin, G.: J. Bone Jt. Surg. **32 A,** 363 (1950)
27. Ricklin, P., Rüttimann, A., del Buono, M. S.: Meniscus lesions. Practical Problems of Clinical Diagnosis, Arthrography and Therapy. Stuttgart: Thieme 1971

28. Roberts, E. M., Metcalf, A.: Mechanical analysis of kicking, medicine and sport: Biomechanics I. 1st. Int. Seminar Zürich 1967. (Ed. Jokl, E.) Basel, New York: Karger 1968
29. Roberts, I. M.: The Surgical Knee. Surg. Clin. N. Amer. **54,** 1313 (1974)
30. Slocum, D. B., Larsen, R. L.: J. Bone Jt. Surg. **50A,** 226 (1968)
31. Slocum, D. B.: J. Bone Jt. Surg. **50A,** 211 (1968)
32. Smillie, I. S.: Injuries of the Knee Joint. Edinburgh–London: Livingstone 1970
33. Smillie, I. S.: Diseases of the Knee Joint. Edinburg–London: Livingstone 1974 Churchill Livingstone 1974
34. Trillat, A., Dejour, H., Couette, A.: Rev. Chir. orthop. **50,** 813 (1964)
35. Trillat, A., Dejour, H.: Rev. Chir. orthop. **53,** 331 (1967)
36. Trillat, A., Dejour, H., Bousquet, G.: Lyon: Simep éditions 1971
37. Trillat, A., Ficat, P.: Rev. Chir. orthop. **58,** Supple. 132 (1972)
38. Winkelmann, B.: Meniskusschaden beim Sportler. 24. Sportärztekongreß in Würzburg, 14.–17. Oktober 1971
39. Zippel, H.: Meniskusverletzungen und Meniskusschäden. Leipzig: Johann Ambrosius Barth 1973

Translation from the German: Die Rotationsstabilität am Kniegelenk. In: Bandverletzungen am Knie, 3. Reisensburger Workshop zur klinischen Unfallchirurgie, edited by C. Burri and A. Rüter. In: Hefte zur Unfallheilkunde, Vol. 125 (1975). © Springer-Verlag 1975.

The Treatment of Unstable Knees

G. Helbing, A. Rüter, and C. Burri

Acute knee ligament injuries may be managed operatively or nonoperatively. Unless there are specific medical contraindications, however, all acute knee ligament ruptures in our clinic are treated surgically. Tears affecting the ligaments alone are sutured and bony avulsions are reinserted with screws or transossous wire sutures. The aim is to restore the function of the knee to an exact anatomic reconstruction.

Most authorities agree that chronic instability from old injuries requires surgical repair. Precise anatomic reconstruction is seldom possible and attempts are, therefore, made to imitate the anatomic status and stability by means of reconstructive procedures. There are a varied range of materials available for this, including skin, fascia, tendons or meniscii. Preserved grafts such as homologous or heterologous dura or tendons are available and more recently synthetic substitutes have been used. The choice of a pedicle graft is determined by the location of the ligament injury. The iliotibial band and the biceps femoris tendon are available as local material on the lateral side of the knee, the sartorius, gracilis and semitendinosus tendons as well as the semimembranosus are available on the medial side, and use can be made of the patellar quadriceps tendon as well.

We will attempt to summarize the numerous possibilities for ligament substitution. Details of pedicle grafts, skin, and other materials will be discussed by other authors.

Philipps in 1914 [12] described the anterior advancement of a tendon to stabilize the medial collateral ligament (Fig. 1). Edwards in 1921 described [4] a similar technique where the tendon was left attached distally and the proximal end advanced and sutured as a substitute with the proximal stump being fixed to an adjacent tendon. Helfet in 1963 [6] described a similar procedure in which he shifted the sartorius via a bony canal into a vertical position. This provided not only medial support but also aimed for a dynamic reconstruction.

In the case of a lax medial collateral ligament, Mauck in 1936 [10] advocated the distal transplantation of the insertion. Campbell in 1935 [2] recommended reconstruction using fascia as a ligament substitute, folding a strip of fascia down from the thigh to the tibia and then turning it upward again. Brückner in 1969 [13] devised a method of free transplantation of strips of the patellar tendon. The middle portion of the tendon together with the attached bony origin and

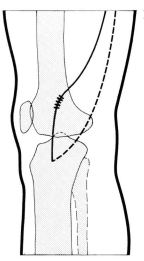

Fig. 1. Anterior shift of the gracilis tendon (Philipps 1914)

insertion from patella and tuberosity is used as a free graft to replace the medial ligament. The same principle can be used on the lateral side. The biceps tendon may also be advanced anteriorly to reconstruct the lateral ligament and this tendon may also be reinforced by the fascia lata also as a pedicle based distally. Edwards recommended using the entire biceps tendon and sewing the proximal stump of the tendon to the tensor fascia to maintain knee flexion [4].

Synthetic materials have also been used with varying degrees of success. These include multiple threads or wires as well as Dacron and Teflon [8], similar to the material used in vascular reconstructions [8].

While the solution is relatively straightforward in isolated collateral ligament injuries, reconstruction of cruciate ligaments is more difficult. There are a wide

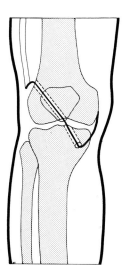

Fig. 2. Repair of the cruciate ligaments with fascia lata (Hey-Groves 1917)

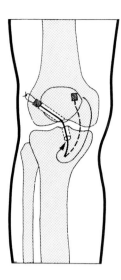

Fig. 3. Repair of the cruciate ligaments with patellar tendon (Brückner 1966)

number of reported techniques indicating that perhaps many of these methods are inadequate. One of the earliest techniques was described by Hey-Groves in 1917 [7] and still continues to be used at present. In this technique a distally pedicled strip of fascia lata is drawn through tunnels drilled in the lateral femoral condyle and medial tibial condyle and finally fixed to the medial side of the femur as a reinforcement for the medial collateral ligament (Fig. 2). O'Donoghue [11] modified this technique by taking a strip of the iliotibial tract, leaving it attached distally close to the head of the fibula, and drawing it through an osseus canal in the head of the tibia and femoral condyle and sewing it back on itself again after it crossed the lateral side of the joint. In this way, the strongest portion of the fascia came into the area of the cruciate ligament and in addition the lateral ligament was reinforced.

Campbell in 1939 [3] used a strip of the medial patellar tendon left attached distally and drawn through a bony tunnel. Jones in 1963 described a similar technique using the middle portion of the tendon into a bony tunnel in the lateral femoral condyle. Brückner in 1969 [1] also described a similar technique (Fig. 3). The Lindemann substitution described in 1950 [9] divides the tendon of semitendinosis or gracilis distally and pulls this through the intercondylar notch inserting it in the area of the tibial tubercle. This produces a reconstruction that is very close to the natural path of the cruciate ligaments (Fig. 4). The tendon of one of these muscles can also serve as a substitute for the cruciate ligaments if it is left attached distally and drawn through corresponding osseus tunnels. Wittek [16] has recommended various methods of using menisci as cruciate substitutes but in our opinion it is unwise to use a healthy meniscus and a damaged meniscus makes a poor substitute.

These techniques must be considered with the risk involved in a major ligament reconstruction and in retrospect, the results have not always justified the

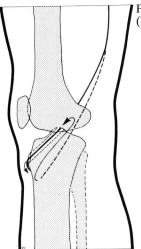

Fig. 4. Repair of the cruciate ligaments with gracilis tendon (Lindemann 1950)

risk. Rotary instability must also be considered. Unfortunately it is frequently overlooked. An extraarticular operation reported by Hauser in 1947 [5] can be used in a combination of rotational and medial instability of the knee (Fig. 5).

The function of a posterior cruciate ligament can be imitated by fixing a strip of the quadriceps tendon left attached at the patella to the medial side of the tibia. The anterior cruciate can be substituted in a similar fashion by taking a strip of the patellar tendon leaving the distal end attached to the tibial tuberosity and attaching the proximal end to the femoral condyle. These two possibilities can be combined in severe cruciate insufficiency and will in addition stabilize the collateral ligament system.

Slocum [14, 15] showed that intrasynovial fascial or tendon grafts stretched over the course of six to twelve months, especially as the patient regained a full

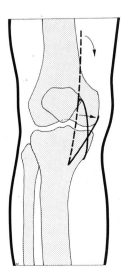

Fig. 5. Extraarticular repair of the cruciate ligaments and collateral ligaments using the quadriceps and patellar tendons (Hauser, 1947)

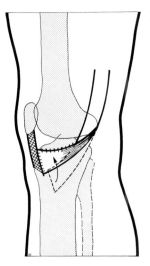

Fig. 6. Pes anserinus transplantation (Slocum 1968)

range of motion. He reported better results from a pes anserina transplantation in 1968 (Fig. 6). The rotary instability caused by injury to the anterior cruciate and medial collateral ligament is eliminated by the mobilization of the distal portion of the pes anserinus and its fixation to the patellar ligament.

This list of the various methods is by no means complete. There are numerous modifications of the principles mentioned. Comments about the respective merits of the procedures are also impossible. The benefit of being able to use a local and often strong tissue as a pedicle replacement is reduced as an undamaged structure becomes impaired by this procedure. Although many methods have been presented it is best to master a few of these techniques and use them well. The functional rehabilitation following ligament reconstruction is of course extremely important.

References

1. Brückner, H.: Eine neue Methode der Kreuzbandplastik. Chirurg 37, 413 (1966)
2. Campbell, W. C.: An operation for repair of the internal and lateral ligament of the knee joint. Surg. Gynec. Obstet. 60, 214 (1935)
3. Campbell, W. C.: Reconstruction of the Ligaments of the Knee. Amer. J. Surg. 43, 473–480 (1939)
4. Edwards, A. H.: Operative procedure suggested for the repair of collateral ligaments of the knee joint. Brit. J. Surg. 8, 266–271 (1921)
5. Hauser, E. D. W.: Extraarticular repair for ruptured collateral and cruciate ligaments. Surg. Gynec. Obstet. 84, 339–345 (1947)
6. Helfet, A. J.: The Management of Internal Derangements of the Knee Joint. London: Pitman 1963
7. Hey-Groves, E. W.: Operation for repair of the cruciate ligaments. Lancet 1917 II, 674
8. Jelinek, R., Gruber, P., Siepen, M.: Der plastische Ersatz der Kniegelenksseitenbänder mit Kunststoffarterien. Zbl. Chir. 87, 1037–1040 (1962)

 9. Lindemann, K.: Über den plastischen Ersatz der Kreuzbänder durch gestielte Sehnenverpflanzung. Z. Orthop. **79,** 316 (1950)
10. Mauck, H. P.: A new operative Procedure for instability of the knee. J. Bone Jt. Surg. **18,** 984–990 (1936)
11. O'Donoghue, D. H.: A method for replacement of the anterior cruciate ligament of the knee. J. Bone Jt. Surg. **45 A,** 906 (1963)
12. Philipps, C. E.: The operative treatment of ruptured ligaments. Surg. Gynec. Obstet. **19,** 729–733 (1914)
13. Pietsch, P., et al.: Ergebnisse plastischer Wiederherstellungsoperationen der Kreuz- und Seitenbänder am Kniegelenk bei 80 Patienten. Mschr. Unfallheilk. **72,** 181–196 (1969)
14. Slocum, D. B., Larson, L.: Pes anserinus transplant. A simple surgical procedure for control of rotatory instability of the knee. J. Bone Jt. Surg. **50 A,** 226 (1968)
15. Slocum, D. B. et al.: Late reconstruction of ligamentous injuries of the medial compartment of the knee. Clin. Orthop. **100,** 23–65 (1974)
16. Wittek, A.: Über Verletzungen der Kreuzbänder des Kniegelenks. Dtsch. Z. Chir. **200,** 491 (1927)

Translation from the German: Therapie-Übersicht beim instabilen Knie. In: Bandverletzungen am Knie, 3. Reisensburger Workshop zur klinischen Unfallchirurgie, edited by C. Burri and A. Rüter. In: Hefte zur Unfallheilkunde, Vol. 125 (1975). © Springer-Verlag 1975.

Pedicled Grafts in the Treatment of the Unstable Knee

I. Schneider and J. Rehn

We use pedicled grafts almost exclusively for the replacement of ligaments in the knee. In our opinion they are almost ideal for this purpose [14]. The strong fascia lata, a large selection of tendons, and even the menisci are available. It is surprising that pedicled grafts were described and adopted later than other techniques [5].

This method has two obvious advantages:

1. The graft consists of the patient's own tissue and there is no danger of rejection.
2. The tissue is immediately accessible and a separate operation to obtain it is unnecessary.

Research has revealed what seems to be yet another advantage [6, 16], namely the superior biologic value of pedicled tendon grafts. The reasons for this high biologic value are thought to be: (a) That the tendon with its pedicle is essentially similar in tissue composition to the ligament which is to be replaced. (b) That its blood supply is in part maintained via the pedicle and the intact paratenon and peritenon [2, 3, 11]. The ingrowth of new capillaries is much quicker and more profuse than in the case of free grafts.

The need to preserve the point of attachment of the pedicled graft may be both an advantage and a disadvantage. Technically, the surgeon's task is certainly easier if fixation is necessary at one end only. The graft can easily be applied under the desired degree of initial tension. On the other hand, there is only one operation in which the fixed point of the graft corresponds almost exactly to the original point of attachment of the ligament: transplantation of the biceps femoris tendon to replace the lateral ligament (Fig. 11). In all the other operations the point of fixation is some distance from the original point of attachment. As the points of origin and insertion of the ligaments are of great relevance to their mechanical function, this must be regarded as a disadvantage. In some instances the grafts can be led through holes drilled in the bone to bring them as close as possible to their ideal point of attachment. This is essential when replacing the cruciate ligaments. However, it is not possible to reproduce the fan-shaped attachment of a ligament — an arrangement which allows different sectors of the ligament to take the strain as the joint moves.

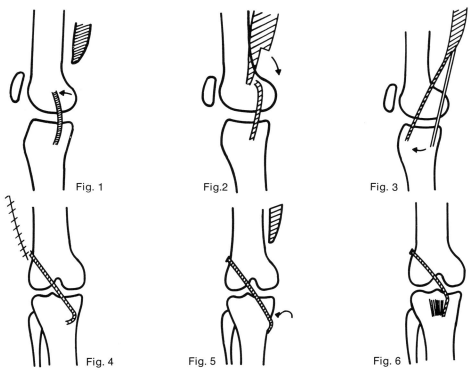

Fig. 1. Gracilis transplantation − Heller
Fig. 2. Adductor magnus transplantation − Salem
Fig. 3. Gracilis or semitendinosus transplantation − Payr
Fig. 4. Fascial transplantation − Hey-Groves
Fig. 5. Gracilis or semitendinosus transplantation − Hey-Groves
Fig. 6. Transplantation of the medial portion of the patellar ligament − Brückner

Pedicled tendon graft operations can be classified into static (Figs. 1, 2, 4, 5, 6, 10, 11) and dynamic (Figs. 3, 7, 8, 9), depending whether the tendon is detached from its muscle belly or whether it is left in continuity with the latter, so that its functional adaptability depends on the contractile power of the muscle. Previous writers have not expressed any clear preference for either of these two options.

Insufficient attention has been paid to the adverse mechanical consequences which may arise from transplantation of whole tendons or parts of tendons. Such possibilities must be borne in mind, especially in operations where the patellar tendon is utilized (Brückner transplantation, Roux-Hauser transplantation) [10] (Figs. 6 and 9) because arthrosis of the patellofemoral joint may result.

A considerable variety of reconstructive operations for repair of the medial ligament by pedicled grafts has been advocated. Pedicled grafts of fascia lata are now seldom used. The tendons which can be employed include the adductor magnus [15] (Fig. 2), gracilis, sartorius, and semitendinosus. Our experience is

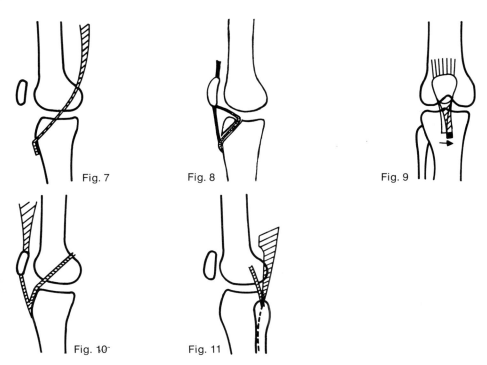

Fig. 7. Gracilis transplantation — Lindemann
Fig. 8. "Dynamic ligament" — Augustine
Fig. 9. Medialization of the patellar ligament — Roux-Hauser
Fig. 10. Transplantation of the central portion of the patellar ligament — Jones
Fig. 11. Biceps tendon transplantation — Krömer

Table 1. Medial ligament repair

Number	Method	Laxity of ligament	Restriction of movement
32	Heller Payr (Figs. 1 and 3)	9	2

based on the use of the gracilis, sartorius, and semitendinosus tendons, both by the static (Fig. 1) and the dynamic principle (Fig. 3). If there are still any remnants of the ligament capable of being reunited, we transfer the semitendinosus or gracilis tendon so that it coincides with the course of the ligament, with the object of conferring extra stability through its active muscular contraction.

When the medial ligament has to be completely replaced, we divide the gracilis or semitendinosus tendon from its muscle belly and pass the cut end through a drill hole in the bone at the original point of insertion of the ligament on the condyle of the femur. The tendon is sutured to itself with Dexon or Mersilene sutures. It is difficult to compare the two methods that we use, because the indications for them are not the same. Little reliance can be placed on patients' subjective statements, because desire for compensation and similar considerations are potent incentives in our trades union practice. Out of 32 medial ligament repairs performed between 1970 and 1972 some laxity of the medial ligament was still demonstrable in nine patients, but it was adequately compensated by tensing the muscles. Some restriction of movement persisted in two of the cases.

Table 2. Lateral ligament

Number	Method	Laxity of ligament	Restriction of movement
7	Krömer (Fig. 11)	0	0

The method of choice for replacing the lateral ligament of the knee has proved to be the pedicled biceps tendon graft [8] (Fig. 11). The biceps tendon is divided longitudinally and half of it is separated from its muscle belly but left attached to its point of insertion on the head of the fibula. Its upper end is then passed through a hole drilled in the lateral epicondyle of the femur and sutured to itself.

Repair of the lateral ligament has been performed in seven patients. In all cases firm ligamentous attachment was achieved and the mobility of the joint was not impaired.

Table 3. Posterior cruciate ligament repair

Number	Method	Laxity of ligament	Restriction of movement
2	Lindemann	2	1

Table 4. Anterior cruciate ligament repair (combined with medial ligament repair)

Number	Method	Laxity of ligament	Restriction of movement
11	Lindemann (Fig. 7)	3	2

The techniques for pedicled graft repair of the cruciate ligaments are now so numerous that they are not easy to summarize. The static procedures include operations using fascia lata [4, 4a] (Fig. 4), parts of the patellar tendon [1, 7] (Figs. 6 and 10), the semitendinosus and gracilis tendons (Fig. 5), and even portions of the medial meniscus detached by trauma [12, 17]. In addition there are dynamic procedures utilizing the gracilis and semitendinosus tendons [9, 13] (Fig. 7) or the patellar tendon [10] (Figs. 8 and 9).

We have no experience in using the meniscus or of Hey-Groves' technique of pedicled fascia grafts. From 1970 to 1972 we used Lindemann's dynamic operation employing the gracilis, semitendinosus or sartorius tendons, and in recent years we have adopted the Jones and Brückner transplantation techniques, using portions of the patellar or quadriceps tendons.

From 1970 to 1972 we followed up in all 31 cases of cruciate ligament injury without avulsion of the bony attachment. Of these 20 were complicated by medial ligament injury. Only in six cases was there an isolated rupture of the anterior cruciate ligament. Rupture of the posterior cruciate ligament, which according to the literature is extremely rare, occurred in three instances and was combined with rupture of the lateral ligament. Late reconstruction of the cruciates was necessary in 13 cases. All the cases reviewed here were operated upon by the technique of dynamic ligament transplantation described by Lindemann in 1950.

The technique of biceps tendon replacement advocated in the literature for rupture of the posterior cruciate was impracticable; because such injuries were accompanied by rupture of the lateral ligament and the biceps tendon was needed to replace the latter. Replacement by the gracilis tendon was tried in two cases but was not satisfactory. The posterior drawer sign remained positive.

Repair of the anterior cruciate was carried out in 11 cases, combined in every instance with replacement of the medial ligament. Good results were obtained in eight cases. Symptomatically the patients were satisfied, with the knee in flexion and the hamstrings tensed, the anterior and posterior drawer signs could no longer be elicited. The other three patients had definite muscle wasting and the anterior drawer sign was still positive. The medial ligament transposition was not secure and the subjective results were unsatisfactory. A good result from repair of the anterior cruciate combined with replacement of the medial ligament will not be obtained unless the integrity of the medial ligament is successfully restored.

References

1. Brückner, H.: Eine neue Methode der Kreuzbandplastik. Chirurg **37**, 413 (1966)
2. Buck, R. G.: Regeneration of tendon. J. Path. Bact. **66**, 1 (1953)
3. Davidsson, L.: Über die subcutanen Sehnenrupturen und die Regeneration der Sehne. Ann. Chir. Gynaec. Fenn. **45**, Suppl. 6, 1 (1956)
4. Hey-Groves, E. W.: Operation for repair of the crucial ligaments. Lancet **1917 II**, 674
4a. Hey-Groves, E. W.: The crucial ligaments of the knee joint: Their function, rupture and the operative treatment of the same. Brit. J. Surg. **7**, 505 (1920)
5. Hierholzer, G., Labitzke, R.: Die Verwendung gestielter Transplantate bei Bandverletzungen. Acta traumatol. **2**, 73–77 (1973)
6. Jokinen, T.: Tensile strength of the whole-thickness skin graft used of the replacement of tendon and ligament defects. Acta Orthop. Scand. **28**, Suppl. 36 (1958)
7. Jones, K. G.: Reconstruction of the anterior cruciate ligament. J. Bone Jt. Surg. **45A**, 925 (1963)
8. Krömer, K.: Zur operativen Behandlung der Seitenbandrisse des Kniegelenkes. Chirurg **34**, 273 (1963)
9. Lindemann, K.: Über den plastischen Ersatz der Kreuzbänder durch gestielte Sehnenverpflanzung. Z. Orthop. **79**, 316 (1950)
10. Matter, P., Burri, C., Rüedi, Th.: Spätzustände nach sofort und sekundär versorgter unhappy triad. Z. Unfallmed. Berufskr. **63**, 34–46 (1970)
11. Närvi, E. J.: Beiträge zur Kenntnis der Sehnenregeneration und Behandlung der Sehnenrupturen, insbesondere im Gebiet der synovialen Scheiden. Acta chir. scand. **60**, 1 (1926)

12. Niederecker, K.: Spätresultate bei Kreuzbandplastik aus einem Meniskus. Chirurg **33,** 88 (1962)
13. Rathke, F. W.: Die gestielte Sehne als plastischer Ersatz der Kreuzbänder. Z. Orthop. **86,** 29 (1955)
14. Rehn, J.: Bandverletzungen des Kniegelenkes. Z. Orthop. **111,** 359–363 (1973)
15. Salem, C.: Zur operativen Therapie veralteter Knieseitenbandrisse. Chirurg **34,** 27 (1963)
16. Salomon, A.: Untersuchungen über die Transplantation verschiedenartiger Gewebe in Sehnendefekte. Langenbecks Arch. Chir. **114,** 523 (1920)
17. Weigert, M., Gronert, H.-J.: Kniebandnaht – Kniebandplastik. Arch. orthop. Unfall-Chir. **72,** 253–271 (1972)

Translation from the German: Gestielte Transplantate in der Behandlung des instabilen Knies. In: Bandverletzungen am Knie, 3. Reisensburger Workshop zur klinischen Unfallchirurgie, edited by C. Burri and A. Rüter. In: Hefte zur Unfallheilkunde, Vol. 125 (1975). © Springer-Verlag 1975.

Free Autologous Skin Grafts in the Treatment of the Unstable Knee

J. Müller, H. Willenegger, and D. Terbrüggen

Skin, fascia, and tendon are this tissues most commonly used as free autologous grafts for replacing the ligaments of the knee. We have little experience in the use of fascial and tendon grafts for this purpose, but for 20 years we have regularly employed autologous skin for the replacement or reinforcement of ligaments. We can therefore speak with some competence on the use of autologous skin as a material for grafts. In this contribution we shall, therefore, confine our remarks to the replacement of knee ligaments with autologous skin.

Between 1961 and 1972 strips of fresh autologous corium were used in 62 cases for direct replacement of the collateral ligaments or the anterior cruciate ligament. Holes are drilled in the bones and the strip is passed through them and pulled tight. Its free ends are then fixed to one another (Table 1).

Table 1. Ligament replacement by free autologous corium strips

Medial ligament alone	18	
+ suture of meniscus	6	
+ meniscectomy	3	27
Lateral ligament		6
Cruciate ligament		7
Combined injuries:		
– anterior cruciate + medial ligament		
(without meniscus injury)	9	
– unhappy triad	13	22
		62

Pathophysiology

The idea which led us to choose this material came from the early studies of Loewe, Rehn, Lexer and Enderlin. These workers established that when strips of autologous skin fixed in tension are used for repair of the abdominal wall or the medial ligament of the knee they will undergo transformation into dense sheets of tendon tissue within 6–10 weeks. As long as 60–70 years ago Enderlin studied the healing process in transplants of autologous skin and demonstrated by means of injection preparations that anastomoses between the capillaries of the host tissue and those of the autologous skin transplant were formed within two days. Later studies have shown that such vascular anastomoses may appear within a few hours. Lymphatic anastomoses have been demonstrated as early as five days afterwards.

Autologous skin transplants offer an opportunity of securing integral healing or assimilation of tissues. Among our own patients there was one instance in which a strip of corium, inserted under tension, showed full thickness revascularization and massive collagen formation with orientated fiber bundles within *one* week (bioptic material). From the investigations carried out to date it is reasonable to conclude that strips of fresh autologous corium kept under tension will heal, at least in part, by a process of assimilation and not solely by mere substitution, as is the case when preserved skin is used. There can be no doubt that as regards its readiness to undergo assimilation and substitution, fresh autologous skin is far superior to any bradytrophic tissues such as fascia, tendon, dura, etc.

After completion of the first phase of healing (vascularization) the functional demands (tensional stresses) imposed on what was originally a highly differentiated covering tissue cause it to develop into young connective tissue, rich in nuclei and blood vessels, while at the same time the accessory structures of the skin (sebaceous and sweat glands, hair follicles, etc.) disappear. The fiber bundles, which originally ran in various directions and were arranged in several layers, are converted by the formative stimulus of tensional stress into bundles

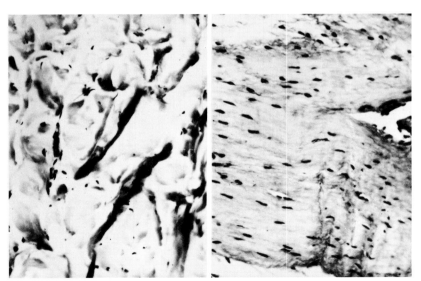

Fig. 1. Photograph of normal skin as seen through the light microscope. The collagen fabrils run in different directions and lie at several levels in relation to one another. Biopsy from the anterior cruciate ligament 11 months after reconstruction with autologous corium (specimen taken during a second operation). All the collagen fibrils run parallel and in the same direction. This photomicrograph shows no difference from normal tendon tissue

uniformly orientated in the same direction, in other words into genuine tendinous tissue (Fig. 1).

Provided that the implanted skin remains under tension, the epidermal accessory structures will usually undergo complete regression. The process of conversion usually takes about three months. Apart from occasional vestiges of gland ducts, we have never found any epidermal remnants. This holds true, however, only if the implant is kept under adequate tension, otherwise there is some danger that epidermoid cysts may develop (Peer-Paddock, Meier). The mechanical properties of fresh corium offer a further advantage, namely that its resistance to tearing is twice that of fascia. Should wound infection occur, implants of autologous corium display much better healing powers than implants of more inert tissues, be they autologous or homologous or bradyotrophic. Rehn pointed out this fact over 50 years ago and we can confirm it from our own cases. Finally, we emphasize that autologous skin is available in every situation and can be excised without difficulty. It does not entail any expensive collection or preservation procedures and it is always available in adequate amounts.

Surgical Techniques

Collection of Skin: As sources of corium we have used the lateral part of the buttock, the lateral side of the thigh or, more recently, the surgical wound itself. We take a strip of skin approximately 2 cm wide and 12–15 cm long. The attached subcutaneous tissue is removed with scissors, and the epithelial layer is merely scraped off with a sharp scalpel. The rectangle of skin thus dissected is then split longitudinally by two or three cuts but left in continuity, so as to produce the longest possible corium strip (Fig. 2). It is then placed in polybactrin solution until required for reimplantation.

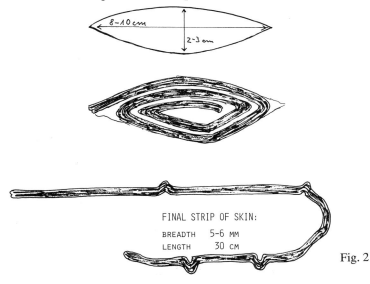

FINAL STRIP OF SKIN:

BREADTH   5-6 MM

LENGTH   30 CM

Fig. 2

Replacement of Collateral Ligaments: To reconstruct the collateral ligaments horizontal drillholes are made in the femoral and tibial condyles, running antero-posteriorly through the bone at the insertions of the ligaments. The corium strip, resembling a shoelace in appearance, is passed through so as to make a circle and then a figure of eight as well (Fig. 3). With associated meniscus injuries, we feel that a peripherally torn but otherwise intact meniscus should not be removed. We advocate meniscectomy only when it is impracticable to suture the meniscus. For extensive marginal tears suturing of the meniscus is combined with replacement of the medial ligament. This is done by drawing the circularly arranged skin strip with its lateral and dorsal loop directly through the base of the medial meniscus (Fig. 4). In this way the meniscus is reattached to the new medial ligament, thus reproducing its natural attachment to the original ligament. Postoperatively, all patients who have undergone reinforcement or replacement of the medial or lateral ligament are immobilized for 6−8 weeks in plaster with the knee flexed 10°−15°. The patient is allowed to put weight on the leg from the start, a measure which ensures some degree of quadriceps training (Tables 2 and 3).

Table 2. Follow-up of 5 cases of replacement of the *lateral* ligament showed the following results 3−14 years postoperatively

Lateral ligament	5
− ligaments equally secure in both knees	3
− impairment of function	0
− adduction laxity: mild	1
severe	1
− muscle atrophy	2
− symptoms: susceptibility to weather changes	1
sensations of weakness in the leg	2
interference with walking	1
− sport: as before the operation	3
no longer possible	2
− reoperation	1

Table 3. Follow-up of cases of replacement of the *medial* ligament (including meniscus suture) showed the following results 3−14 years postoperatively

Medial ligament	27
− ligaments equally secure in both knees	21
− functional impairment (flexion − 10°)	4
(flexion − 20°)	2
− abduction laxity: mild	6
severe	2
− meniscus signs	0
− muscle atrophy	5
− symptoms: susceptibility to weather changes	3
− sensations of weakness in the leg	7
interference with walking	2
− sport: as before the operation	16
no longer possible	6
− reoperation	1

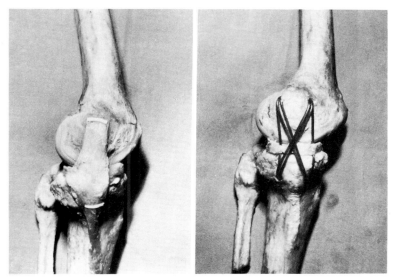

Fig. 3. Diagram of the medial ligament. The ligament is inserted along a line running parallel to the joint surface. This line is marked. The second diagram shows how the medial ligament is replaced by a strip of corium, the meniscus being secured at the same time

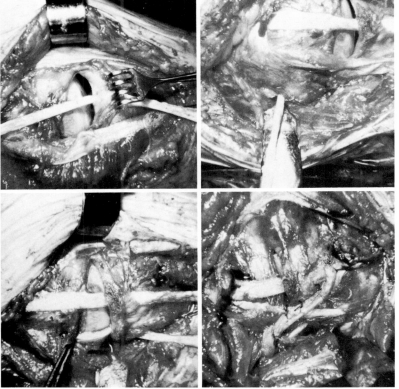

Fig. 4. B. L., 21 years, ski accident. Total rupture of the medial ligament on the left side. Avulsion of meniscus. Repair with autologous corium. Surgical technique

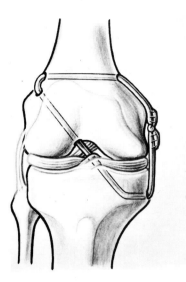

Fig. 5. Replacement of the anterior cruciate ligament with a strip of corium (diagrammatic). A modification of Hey-Groves' operation

Replacement of the Anterior Cruciate Ligament and Treatment of Combined Injuries: To replace the anterior cruciate ligament by a graft, we use a modified Hey-Groves procedure. The skin is drawn through drill holes so that the free ends of the corium strips can be sutured to one another on the medial side at a point outside their transosseous anchorage (Fig. 5). When replacing the anterior cruciate ligament it is essential to ensure that the transosseous anchorage at the distal end of the femur is located at the exact position of the original insertion of the ligament. The meniscus lesion so commonly associated with these combined injuries is dealt with at the same time as the replacement of the medial ligament. Whenever possible we strive to preserve an intact meniscus, if it has been avulsed only at its periphery. In our own series, suture of the meniscus was feasible in 11 cases of this kind.

Even in cases with extensive marginal tears, suture of the meniscus was combined with repair of the medial ligament as described above. Postoperatively, all patients, whether they had undergone cruciate ligament replacement alone or

Table 4. Late results after isolated replacement of anterior cruciate ligament

Anterior cruciate ligament	6
– functional impairment	0
– adduction or abduction laxity: mild	1
severe	0
– forward drawer sign: mild	5
severe	1
– muscle atrophy	3
– symptoms: susceptibility to weather changes	1
sensations of weakness in the leg	2
interference with walking	1
– sport: as before the operation	3
no longer possible	3
– reoperation	0

Table 5. Late results after combined injuries

Combined injuries	22
− functional impairment (flexion − 10°)	5
(flexion − 20°)	4
− ligaments equally secure in both knees	11
− adduction or abduction laxity: mild	7
severe	4
− rotational instability: mild	7
severe	3
− drawer sign: mild	11
severe	5
− muscle atrophy	9
− symptoms: susceptibility to weather changes	7
sensations of weakness in the leg	6
interference with walking	4
− sport: as before the operation	11
no longer possible	9
− reoperation	3

operations for repair of combined injuries (medial ligament and anterior cruciate) were immobilized in a plaster for an average of 10−12 weeks with the knee flexed 10°−15°. We permit patients in plaster to put full weight on the leg. These patients with cruciate repairs alone and combined injuries have been followed up for 3−14 years. The late results for isolated anterior replacement are as follows:

In summary, our series comprises 62 cases from the years 1969−1972, in which ligaments were directly replaced with fresh autologous corium. All these cases have been followed up. Among them were 15 late reconstructions carried out 3 months to 22 years after the accident and 47 repairs carried out on an acute basis. The outcome in all 62 cases as assessed by subjective and objective criteria can be summarized as follows:

Very good	20
Good	34
Poor	8
	62

The best results were obtained on the medial ligament with full restoration of ligament stability in 21 out of 27 cases.

We are convinced that it is better to master a single technique for transplant replacement of ligaments than to experiment with a variety of techniques.

References

Bruck, H.: Arch. klin. Chir. **303,** 277 (1973).
Janik, B.: Kreuzbandverletzungen des Kniegelenkes. Berlin: Walter de Gruyter 1955
Lezius, R.: Chirurg, **17/18,** 132 (1947)
Loewe, H.: Münch. med. Wschr. **24,** 1320 (1912)

Müller, J.: Mschr. Unfallheilk. **110,** 78 (1971)

Müller, J., Willenegger, H., Schuster, K.: Z. Unfallmed. Berufskr. **70,** 23 (1970)

Peer-Paddock, J. N.: Arch. Surg. **34,** 268 (1937)

Rehn, E.: Arch. klin. Chir. **112,** 622 (1919)

Stengel, H.: Chirurg **27,** 70 (1956)

Willenegger, H.: Arch. klin. Chir. **308,** 954 (1964)

Willenegger, H., Baltensperger, A.: Helv. chir. Acta **34,** 75 (1967)

Willenegger, H., Müller, J., Klumpp, E., Al-Haddad, H.: Ligament repair in recent and longstanding knee injuries by autogenous skin graft. In: Injuries of the Ligaments and Their Repair. Chapchal, G. (ed.). Stuttgart, Thieme, 1977

Translation from the German: Freie autologe Transplantate in der Behandlung des instabilen Knies. In: Bandverletzungen am Knie, 3. Reisensburger Workshop, edited by C. Burri and A. Rüter. In: Hefte zur Unfallheilkunde, Vol. 125 (1975). ©Springer-Verlag 1975.

The Acute Cartilage Injury

Arthroscopy in Articular Cartilage Injury

W. Glinz

The recognition of lesions affecting only articular cartilage is undoubtedly one of the most difficult diagnostic problems in knee joint injuries. The mechanism of injury and the clinical examination may suggest such a diagnosis but do not allow an accurate assessment of the nature of the injury nor its extent. Plain-X-rays are usually normal and arthrography is only helpful when carried out by an experienced examiner.

Arthroscopy of the knee was performed as early as 1918 by Takagi in Toyko [7] and in 1921 by Bircher [1]. It permits direct observation of all cartilage surfaces of the knee joint. The extent and the nature of the cartilage lesion can be clearly determined and a plan of treatment established. Endoscopic operations can also be performed such as the removal of loose bodies or the resection of localized areas of damaged articular or semilunar cartilage.

Arthroscopy of the knee is coming into wider use and general acceptance [2, 3, 5, 6, 8, 9]. This technique however is an extremely complex method of examination and its advantages can be fully realized only in the hands of a practiced examiner. Arthroscopy is indicated when other methods have failed to produce sufficient information.

Examination Technique

We use a cold light arthroscope with flexible fiber-optics (Stortz, Tuttlingen, West Germany). The instrument with an advanced view optic has an angle of vision of 30°. It is inserted into the joint through the shaft of the trocar, diameter 4.5 mm. (Fig. 1). Biopsy forceps with a direct view optic can also be used through the same shaft. Trocars with smaller diameters are also available, but seem to offer no advantages.

Arthroscopy is carried out under general anesthetic. The joint can then be moved without restriction. Selective biopsies produce no difficulty The risk of articular cartilage injury with an unexpected movement of the patient is eliminated. Most examinations are done in the outpatient department with the

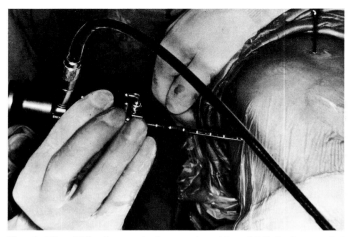

Fig. 1. The 30° advanced view optic with cold light inserted through a flexible fiber-optic cord is inserted into the knee joint

patient returning home the same evening. Arthroscopy requires strictly aseptic conditions and is performed in the operating theatre. A pneumatic tourniquet is used and the knee is prepared and draped as for an arthrotomy. Normal saline is introduced into the suprapatellar pouch, the trocar is inserted into the joint through a stab wound, the medial joint compartment normally being inspected from a point just lateral to the patellar tendon and the lateral joint compartment from a medial insertion. The deep surface of the patella can be inspected from either approach or through a separate stab wound in the superolateral recess.

Morbidity Rate and Complications

The main advantage of arthroscopy over arthrotomy is the low morbidity rate. The examination causes practically no quadriceps inhibition. Most patients return to work one to two days following the examination.

Infection is the most feared complication. In our series of 208 arthroscopies, we have not had any significant complications. According to the literature, the risk of infection is slight [6, 8].

Case Material

In the past three years we have performed arthroscopies on 208 patients. Almost all are traumatic lesions. Seventy-five patients showed cartilage injury.

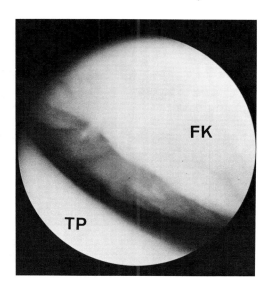

Fig. 2. Ulcer craters on the medial femoral condyle (FK – femoral condyle TP tibial plateau)

Only 25 of these were suspected as a result of history and clinical examination. Articular cartilage injury in our series is the second most frequent arthroscopic diagnosis. It is exceeded only by meniscal injury.

Articular Cartilage Injury of Femoral Condyles or Tibial Plateaus

Unlike Wruhs we feel that arthroscopy is seldom indicated in recent trauma [3]. This avoids many unnecessary and avoidable examinations. If there is a cartilage injury with a free fragment suspected, then an arthroscopic examination may be indicated in the acutely injured knee.

A better time for arthroscopy is a few weeks postinjury when the acute affects of the trauma have subsided. Frequently the examination is carried out much later for residual posttraumatic symptoms. Arthroscopy is also useful in other knee complaints such as locking or effusions when other methods have not established the diagnosis. The surfaces of both femoral condyles and tibial plateaus can be seen almost completely using the 30° advanced view optic. The possible injuries to the cartilage are many and varied. They include simple tears in the articular cartilage, avulsions of portions of cartilage, areas of chondromalacia, flaking or fraying, and even frank ulcers (Fig. 2.)

We differentiate between two main types of posttraumatic prearthrosis findings [4]. The first a localized cartilage injury usually after direct damage and secondly generalized granular changes diffusely scattered in the knee as might be seen after a prolonged hemarthrosis.

Most of our patients had the articular cartilage injury to femoral condyle or tibial plateau. The precise localization was made clinically in only a few cases. Arthroscopy on the other hand, accurately located the site of injury, although an arthrotomy was not indicated in most patients. In acute lesions on weight-bearing surfaces, we recommend mobilization with restricted weight-bearing. Only five patients required an arthrotomy to deal with the articular cartilage lesion. With only one exception, no patients had cartilage injuries resulting from intraarticular fracture. Such a case is usually not a diagnostic problem as the X-rays or clinical examination usually indicate a problem. Our one exception was a patient in whom a lateral meniscal lesion was suspected after a conservatively treated fracture of the lateral tibial plateau. Arthroscopy showed no signs of an injury to the meniscus and to our surprise the articular surfaces of the tibial plateaus were completely healed and intact. However there was extensive cartilage damage to both femoral condyles.

Twenty-three patients had arthroscopy one year following meniscectomy. We noted marked changes in the articular cartilage in 21 of these. The changes were definitely prearthrotic, and X-rays revealed no change. The cartilage changes in these early stages were mostly localized. As expected the articular damage after a meniscectomy is usually situated on the surfaces adjacent to the site of meniscectomy. However cartilage surfaces of other parts of the joint were also frequently involved and in a few patients, we discovered single or multiple areas of damage in the opposite compartment.

Table 1. Prearthrotic Changes after Meniscectomies (21 patients)

Femoral Condyle	– same side	16
Tibial Plateau	– same side	15
Femoral Condyle	– other side	5
Tibial Plateau	– other side	8

The frequent and early damage after meniscectomy has strengthened our belief that this operation is not benign. The loss of the meniscus causes mechanical damage to the articular cartilage of the adjacent surfaces of the femur and tibia. Iatrogenic damage was also clearly identified in a few cases.

Cartilage Damage to the Deep Surface of the Patella

Trauma to the deep surface of the patella and the symptoms of chondromalacia are common. Thirty-eight patients had positive findings in this area. Injuries to the deep surface of the patella are suspected more frequently than those on the femoral condyle or tibial plateau, but often the diagnosis is false. Frequently with a clinical diagnosis of retropatellar damage, we discovered with athroscopy that the articular cartilage was completely intact. It is not easy to diagnose injuries in this area. Chondromalacia is often assumed in cases of unexplained knee complaints as an escape.

The arthroscope allows complete and easy observation of the deep surface of the patella. The examination is carried out through the same incision as for the examination of the medial compartment. If positive findings are present or if the view is insufficient, a superolateral stab wound will allow further visualization. Arthroscopy helps considerably not only in confirming the diagnosis of retropatellar injuries, but also in determining the indications for operative treatment and selecting the operative procedure. We have frequently noted minor changes which do not require surgical intervention. The changes on the deep surface of the patella are varied in our experience. Fraying of the cartilage is frequently seen (Figs. 3, 4, 5).

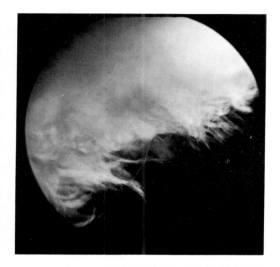

Fig. 3. Articular cartilage injury to the deep surface of the patella with frayed articular cartilage

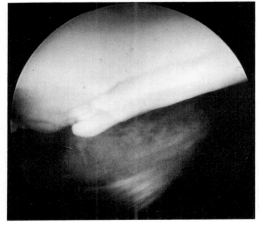

Fig. 4. A traumatic furrow-shaped tear in the articular cartilage of the patella

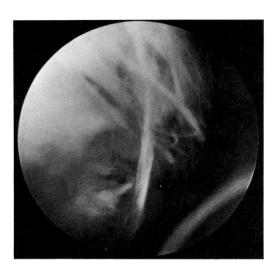

Fig. 5. Frayed articular cartilage around the bed in a case of osteochondritis dissecans

Meniscal Damage Secondary to Changes in Articular Cartilage

Articular cartilage injury and subsequent prearthrosis or even arthrosis often causes mechanical wear of the meniscus. Twenty patients showed such changes. The most usual finding was fraying of the meniscal substances, especially on its free edge. Such changes are not an indication for meniscectomy. The problem would only be worsened by the removal of the buffer between the damaged areas of articular cartilage. Small tears on the free edge (Fig. 6) are not an indication for meniscectomy. Meniscectomy should be reserved for those patients in which there is an actual fissure in the meniscus.

In two of our patients we observed that small detached fragments of articular cartilage had caused considerable damage to the meniscus (Fig. 7).

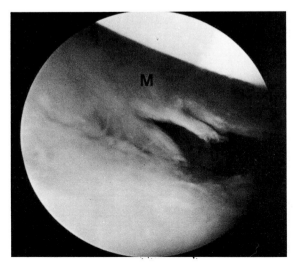

Fig. 6. Damage to the lateral meniscus with small tears on the free edge in a case of severe arthrosis of the knee joint

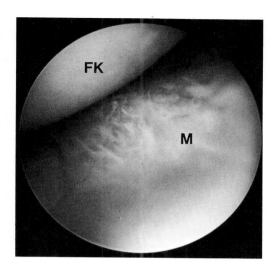

Fig. 7. Injury to the anterior surface of the medial meniscus from small traumatically separated fragments of cartilage which were removed with the help of an arthroscope (M - meniscus, FK — femoral condyle)

Endoscopic Surgery in Cases of Articular Cartilage Injury

Endoscopic operations have the same low morbidity as the purely diagnostic arthroscopy. Such procedures are not easy and should only be done by surgeons practiced in this area. The arthroscope can be used to remove loose bodies or damaged segments of articular cartilage.

Removal of Loose Bodies

Although biopsy forceps can be inserted through the shaft of the scope, the removal of loose bodies with these forceps is practically impossible as the loose body tends to be pushed away by the insertion of the forceps. For this reason, we have given up removing loose bodies by this method.

Small loose bodies that will pass through the shaft of the arthroscope (4.5 mm) can be caught in the far end of the shaft by retracting the optics slightly. The entrapment of the loose body can be checked out through the lens. The optics are then removed and the solution in the joint washes the loose body out through the shaft (Fig. 8). We use special forceps to remove larger loose bodies (Figs. 9 and 10). These are inserted through a small separate incision. The loose body is located and under direct vision the forceps are closed over it. The loose body is then pulled to the joint capsule and the incision in skin and capsule enlarged sufficiently to allow its removal. Fragments of practically any size can be removed in this way. Normally skin sutures are all that is required to close the additional incision.

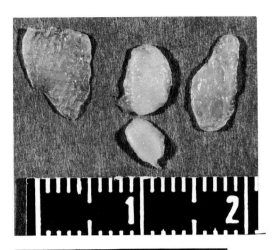

Fig. 8. Such small free-floating fragments can be removed through the shaft of the arthroscope

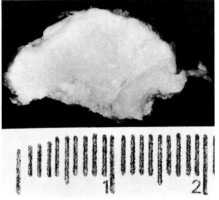

Fig. 9. Larger fragments are trapped under direct observation and removed through a small separate incision

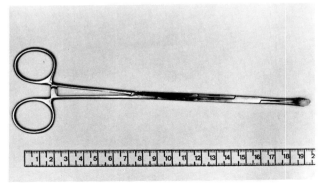

Fig. 10. The special forceps used to remove loose bodies that are larger than 4.5 mm

Removal of Damaged Fragments of Articular Cartilage

Circumscribed damaged fragments of articular cartilage that are raised and flaky can be removed with biopsy forceps during continuous observation through an arthroscope. This will clean out the area of cartilage damage. The procedure is quite practical on small cartilage lesions but needs great patience. Larger areas where debridement is necessary or surfaces where it is difficult to judge the extent of injury are best approached and dealt with by a small arthrotomy. Even in such cases, however, arthroscopy enables us to use the smallest possible operative incision as it is possible to accurately localize the area of damage.

Summary

Arthroscopy has become an important and sometimes an indispensable tool for the diagnosis of articular cartilage damage in the knee. It allows examination of all cartilage surfaces within the knee joint. The examination is carried out under sterile conditions in an operating theatre under general anesthesia. A cold light arthroscope with a 30° advanced view optic is used and is inserted through a trocar with a diameter of 4.5 mm. Most examinations are done in the outpatient department, the rate of morbidity is extremely low. In 208 arthroscopies, mostly posttraumatic cases, 75 patients showed damage to articular cartilage. Only one-third of these had this injury suspected on clinical examination. Arthroscopy is useful in the removal of loose bodies and to a limited extent in the removal or debriding of small circumscribed areas of cartilage damage.

References

1. Bircher, E.: Die Arthroendoskopie. Zbl. Chir. **48,** 1460 (1921)
2. Casscells, S. W.: Arthroscopy of the knee joint. J. Bone Jt. Surg. **53 A,** 287 (1971)
3. Glinz, W.: Arthroscopy in trauma of the knee joint. In: The Knee Joint. Proceedings of the international congress. Rotterdam 1973, **113,** Excerpta Medica, Amsterdam 1974
4. Glinz, W.: Diagnostische Bedeutung der Arthroskopie bei Präarthrosen des Kniegelenkes. Z. Unfallmed. Berufskr. **67,** 260 (1974)
5. Henche, H. R.: Indikation, Technik und Resultate der Arthroskopie nach Traumatisierung des Kniegelenkes. Orthopädie **3,** 178 (1974)
6. Jackson, R. W., Abe, I.: The role of arthroscopy in the management of disorders of the knee. J. Bone Jt. Surg. **54 B,** 310 (1972)
7. Takagi, K.: Practical experiences using Takagi's arthroscope. J. Jap. Orthop. Ass. **22,** 59 (1949)
8. Watanabe, M., Takeda, S., Ikeuchi, H.: Atlas of Arthroscopy. 2nd. ed. Tokyo: Igaku Shoin 1969
9. Wruhs, O.: Die Arthroskopie und Endphotographie zur Diagnostik und Dokumentation von Kniegelenksverletzungen. Wien. med. W. **120,** 126 (1970)
10. Wruhs, O.: Endoskopisch faßbare Veränderungen des Femur-Patellargelenkes. Z. Orthop. **111,** 525 (1973)

Translation from the German: Arthroskopie beim Knorpelschaden des Kniegelenks. In: Knorpelschaden am Knie, 4. Reisensburger Workshop zur klinischen Unfallchirurgie, edited by C. Burri and A. Rüter. In: Hefte zur Unfallheilkunde, Vol. 127 (1976). © Springer Verlag 1976.

Posttraumatic Cartilage Impression of the Femoral Condyles

E. Morscher

Introduction

Posttraumatic knee pain is one of the most difficult differential diagnostic problems facing the traumatologist and orthopaedic surgeon. Fractures, meniscal, and ligamentous lesions are well understood as causes of knee pain. Injuries to the articular surface of the tibia, femoral condyles, or patella may also be the cause of long-lasting and refractory complaints.

Chondromalacia patellae and osteochondral fractures are the most frequently found traumatic cartilage lesions. Osteochondritis if located on the lateral femoral condyle is often a traumatic lesion. In addition to these three types we have in recent years observed changes in articular cartilage which are generally unrecognized but in our opinion are of pathologic significance. This is a cartilage impression usually on the medial femoral condyle and may be responsible for many cases of knee pain.

As Wagner [7] has reported we distinguish between the following types of injury to articular cartilage caused either by direct or indirect contusion.

1. Two-dimensional impressions or depressed fractures – These are real fractures with a fragment depressed into the underlying cancellous bone. The fragment has a characteristic jagged ridge.

2. Resilient cartilage bone impression — These occur only on osteoporotic femoral condyles. After the contusion causes a slight depression, the subchondral bone may remain compressed, while the cartilage itself regains its original shape.

3. Impressions of the articular crest on the femoral condyle — These were only mentioned in passing by Smillie [6] in his classic monograph, "Injuries of the Knee Joint." He noted, especially in female patients with genu recurvatum, that not only is the anterior horn pressed between the condyles of the femur and tibia and thereby injured, but also that a depression may result in the articular cartilage of the femoral condyle.

After observing several cases in which an impression on the medial femoral condyle alone or in combination with other injuries caused knee pain, we felt

that this observation should be reported [Morscher, 3, 4, 5]. Wagner [7] reported thirteen such crest impressions, in his article on "Traumatic Cartilaginous
Injuries of the Knee Joint."

Case Material

We have observed 43 impressions on the femoral condyle which we have desig-
nated pathologic or posttraumatic. This has occurred as the only finding or as a
primary or secondary finding in other damage to the knee joint. Twenty patients
were men and 23 were women. The men had an average age of 36 years
(12–62) and the women 30 years (9–46). In 37 cases the medial femoral condyle was affected and the lateral in only six. Twenty-four were found on the right
knee and 19 on the left. All findings reported were operative.

The most obvious mechanism, forced hyperextension, was only found in one-
tenth of the cases. In two-thirds, either direct contusion or indirect trauma to the
affected knee was reported. Only seven patients denied injury.

Table 1. Case Material — Impressions on the Femoral Condyles

Mechanism of Injury	Only Finding	Primary Finding	Secondary Finding	%
No trauma	2	5	–	16%
Questionable trauma	–	2	–	4.6%
Forced hyperextension	–	3	1	9.3%
Direct contusion	3	7	3	27.9%
Twisting or angulation	2	7	6	34.8%
Other	–	2	–	7.4%
Total	16%	60.5%	23.5%	

Operative Findings

The crest impression on the femoral condyle was diagnosed by us at the time of
arthrotomy. In most cases this impression was the only pathologic finding and,
therefore, the only explanation for the patients, complaints. In other cases the
impression was a secondary finding, however, there appeared to be a pathogenic
connection between the impression and the other lesions. This will be discussed
later.

The crest impressions extended from one to several cms in diameter. In some,
crests were visible and palpable; in others, a shallow depression. When the knee
joint is extended the depression is usually located opposite the contact point
corresponding to the anterior horn of the medial miniscus. The articular cartilage
above the impression exhibits clear, pathologic alterations in the form of soften-

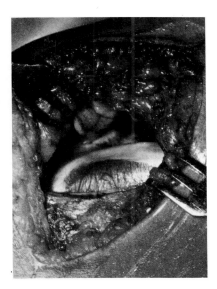

Fig. 1. Typical finding of a cartilaginous impression on the femoral condyle with degenerate alterations of the articular cartilage within the area of the impression and pannus formation

ing, yellowish discoloration, and a dull appearance. Occasionally genuine erosions are observed. The formation of a pannus is considered to be clearly pathologic (Fig. 1). The synovial vascular pannus extends from the cartilage synovial junction towards the impression. The cartilage under the pannus is degenerate.

In many cases chondromalacia of the patella was found in addition to the impression on the medial or lateral femoral condyle. The simultaneous occurrance of chondromalacia patella with other knee joint pathology (e.g., meniscal lesions) is well known. On the other hand, the etiology of chondromalacia is not explicable in all cases and in some patients the localization of the retropatellar softening when the knee joint was flexed corresponded exactly to the point on the articular cartilage across from the impression. This was usually on the medial facet. In these cases it might be assumed that the incongruity of the femoral joint caused by the impression had led to the chondromalacia. Quite often alterations on the anterior horn of the meniscus occur which frequently fit into the impression. The anterior horn of the meniscus sometimes develops degeneration and in other cases a pannus develops as a sign of chronic irritation.

Diagnosis

As mentioned previously, a traumatic cartilaginous impression was only considered a primary diagnosis in a few cases. Usually it was discovered after arthroscopy or arthrotomy and then recognized as the cause of the complaints. Once we realized that this injury was a possible cause of posttraumatic knee pain, it appeared more often as a primary diagnosis.

This lesion should be kept in mind if the injury is the result of a hyperextension trauma, a direct contusion or a twisting injury of the knee, and if there is diffusely

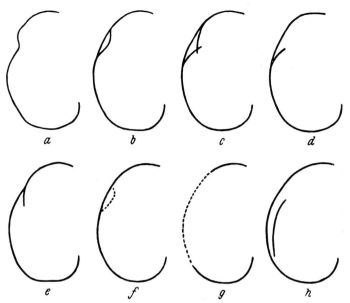

Fig. 2. A–H: Different types of contours in the lateral X-ray of the femoral condyles (from Koehler and Zimmer, 1967)

localized knee pain usually medial without swelling or locking. Local tenderness on the femoral condyle with the knee flexed almost to a right angle is very suspicious. X-rays are not generally helpful since normally there is an impression on the condyle that appears distal to the articular line for the patella. Only in the case of a deeper impression is it justified to suspect a pathologic impression. Koehler and Zimmer [2] distinguish between different types of contours in the lateral X-ray of the femoral condyles (Fig. 2). Examination of our X-rays of patients with and without impressions revealed Type A to be the most frequent.

Pathogenesis and Mechanism of Injury

Viewed laterally the femoral condyles are spiral in shape. The surface of these condyles is, however, not uniform as in a geometric figure but shows physiologically distinct irregularities. The most significant is the line for the patella which as a more or less distinct transverse crest causes the condyle lying above and below to appear as an impression or more accurately a depression. In an extended position it is also very clear that the anterior horns of the meniscus fit into the distal depression (Fig. 3). The question arises, therefore, as to whether these depressions originate during the physiologic development of the knee joint because the anterior horns are pressed into the femoral condyles when completely extended. The pathologically or traumatically incurred crest impressions described here would, therefore, merely correspond to an accent-

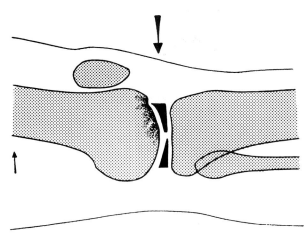

Fig. 3. Traumatic impression on the femoral condyle caused by forced extension of the knee joint. The anterior horn of the meniscus fits exactly into the impression

utation of a basically physiologic. occurrence. The more a knee joint can be hyperextended the greater the force with which the anterior horn of the miniscus can be pressed between the condyles. Therefore, a genu recurvatum which Smillie [6] assumes is the cause of the lesions of the anterior horns is susceptible to an impression of the femoral condyles.

Differential Diagnosis

Serious impressions and other damage to the surface of the condyles are quite often discovered as lesions which accompany meniscus injuries and are caused by displaced meniscal fragments within the interior of the joint [1, 6]. In these cases the meniscal fragment usually fits into the defect in the condyle and is attenuated by the constant crunching of its anterior end in maximum extension. More frequently osteochondral fragments or free cartilaginous fragments are seen.

Discussion

The fact that, when the knee joint is extended the impression on the femoral condyle corresponds to the anterior horn of the medial meniscus opposite it, leaves little doubt as to the pathogenesis of this lesion. Although a hyperextension trauma was reported in only 10% of the cases, it is extremely characteristic of the formation of the femoral condyle impression. The following case summary demonstrates this.

W. S. — Born April 16, 1956:

Case history — In September, 1973 during judo practice the opponent fell directly onto the anterior aspect of the fully extended right knee. Definite hyperextension followed by severe pain and swelling occurred. Because of continuing pain aggravated by stress the patient had to give up athletic activity.

Physical examination on the June 17, 1975, showed a normal gait. There was a normal range of motion without crepitus. Ligaments were stable, there was point tenderness on the medial crest of the medial femoral condyle.

Arthroscopy — June 23, 1975 — The deep surface of the patella was normal. On the medial femoral condyle in the previously observed tender area, a distinct, relatively flat impression was observed about 2 cm in diameter. Within the area of impression the cartilage exhibited yellowish discoloration and was soft. Its surface was partially desquamated. Sporadic smaller cartilaginous villi also projected into the joint. In addition a smaller healed cartilaginous ulcer was discovered. Medially one could observe pannus formation which extended toward the soft cartilage. The menisci were normal.

Arthrotomy — August 5, 1975 — No effusion was present, the deep surface of the patella showed an area of chondromalacia with a small almost puncturelike defect extending to the subchondral bone. There was a flat impression on the femoral condyle. The pannus formation was distinct although not pronounced. The fat pad was partially resected, the impression was lifted, packed with cancellous bone and reinserted. The soft cartilage on the deep surface of the patella was shaved.

Both the degeneration of the cartilaginous surface and the area of the impression and the existence of a pannus which promoted the cartilaginous degeneration support the theory that the observed pathology was not a normal variant of the femoral condyle as described by anatomists.

Treatment

The impressions on the femoral condyles found during arthrotomy were occasionally only a secondry finding and so insignificant that we limited ourselves to removing the vascular pannus. This pannus just as in the case of a primary chronic polyarthritis must be considered pathologic and destructive to articular cartilage. In order to lessen the constant pressure of the anterior horn of the medial meniscus it was removed in some cases.

Massive impressions and those which represented the only pathologic finding in the painful knee should be "re-set." To do this we make a proximal cortical window from the outer surface of the affected femoral condyle with a small sharp curette a passage is made down to the impression and from this point using either a periosteal elevator or punch, the impression is lifted from the subchondral side. The defect in the cancellous bone is then packed with cancellous graft. Full extension and weight-bearing is restricted for six weeks following the procedure.

Conclusions

In the cases involving degenerative cartilage alterations and pannus formation the impression on the medial or lateral femoral condyle is undoubtedly a pathologic finding. This can be explained most easily as the result of hyperextension or direct contusion of the knee joint. The majority of those diagnosed by us either as the only pathologic finding or as a secondary finding were discovered by accident. In many cases the impression could be considered a cause of a chondromalacia localized on the medial facet of the patella. The diagnosis of an impression on the medial femoral condyle is not easy since irregularities of the subchondral bony layer on the medial femoral condyle occur physiologically. The lesion is easily seen at arthroscopy. It should be sought during every arthrotomy.

References

1. Bonnin, J. G.: Osteochondritis dissecans and torn lateral meniscus, J. Bone Jt. Surg. **33,** 380 (1946)
2. Koehler, A., Zimmer, E. A.: Grenzen des Normalen und Anfänge des Pathologischen im Röntgenbild des Skeletts, Stuttgart: Thieme 1967
3. Morscher, E.: Traumatische Knorpel-Knochenläsionen am Kniegelenk. Orthop. Praxis **6,** 31 (1970)
4. Morscher, E. Pfeiffer, K. M.: Spätschäden nach Knorpel- und Knochenimpressionen am Kniegelenk. Z. Unfallmed. Berufskr. **1,** 47 (1970)
5. Morscher E.: Cartilage-Bone Lesions of the Knee Joint. Reconstr. Surg. Traumat. **12,** 2 (1971)
6. Smillie, I. S.: Injuries of the Knee Joint, 4th ed. Edinburgh, London: Livingstone 1970
7. Wagner, H.: Traumatische Knorpelschäden des Kniegelenkes. Orthopäde **3,** 208 (1974)

Translation from the German: Traumatische Knorpelimpression an den Femurcondylen. In: Knorpelschaden am Knie, 4. Reisensburger Workshop zur klinischen Unfallchirurgie, edited by C. Burri and A. Rüter. In: Hefte zur Unfallheilkunde, Vol. 127 (1976).
© Springer-Verlag 1976.

The Isolated Shear Injury to Articular Cartilage

R. Ganz

Injuries to the articular cartilage not affecting the underlying subchondral bone are frequently observed as small multiple abrasions in cases of dislocations or subluxation. Good examples would be the dome of the talus or the head of the femur. Impressions on the articular cartilage without subchondral damage are frequent and often take the form of star-shaped marks, particularly after a contusion to the articular surface of the patella. In contrast, large areas of cartilage shorn-off without attached subchondral bone are seldom seen. They have only been described in knee joints [4, 7, 10].

Because of the close connection between the cartilage and subchondral bone osteochondral avulsions are the rule. To allow shear injury of cartilage alone the corresponding articular surfaces must be so tightly pressed together that, as the joint moves, no sliding movement is possible. Such a situation can be imagined in the knee when there is forced rotation with a slightly flexed knee under maximal pressure. The area of cartilage under such stress must be at a specific size or an osteochondral fracture would be more probable. Such specific conditions can be confirmed in two out of five cases of shear injuries to cartilage. In the case of two ski racers, the series of movements in the fall were very complex. It is most probable that the initial portion of the fall when the skier was thrown off his course was responsible for the cartilage injury. In one other case the shearing of an extensive area of cartilage from the lateral femoral condyle occurred in connection with a traumatic dislocation of the patella.

Previous injuries to articular cartilage may play a role. Such damage seems likely in the knees of high-performance athletes who through repeated micro-trauma have disturbed the structure of the cartilage. Even if macroscopic changes are not observed during arthrotomy, ruptures in the tangential layer of collagen fibres is likely. Such factors, however, can be excluded in the case of extensive shear injury as the result of the patellar dislocation in a 11-year-old girl (Fig. 1). Early diagnosis is essential for a good long term prognosis [6]. X-rays do not provide any help as the lesion affects only the articular cartilage. The clinical examination is the key. Errors in diagnosis such as meniscal or ligamentous injuries are easy to make in this type of accident [3, 5, 6, 9]. Consequently in three out of the five cases diagnosis was delayed until recurrent symptoms and disability forced an arthrotomy.

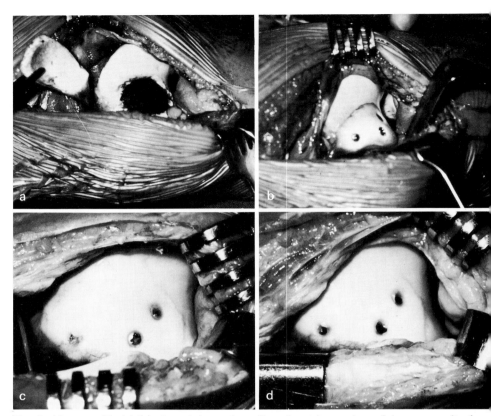

Fig. 1. 11-year-old girl (a) shear injury of cartilage from femoral condyle as a result of patellar dislocation, (b) Fixation with small A. O. screws, (c and d) Appearance three months later. The fragment of cartilage has healed

In the three cases undergoing delayed arthrotomy, the detached cartilage had been damaged by joint motion and was removed. As there was no sign of fresh bleeding on the subchondral bone, a forage was carried out to promote granulation and fibrocartilage formation (Fig. 2) [7, 8, 10]. The postoperative treatment consisted of early movement with a cautious degree of pressure. In one case, the avulsion of a large flap of regenerated fibrocartilage made a further operation necessary.

In the two other cases arthrotomy was done immediately following injury. In both cases there was an extensive lesion and the free fragment of cartilage showed no changes. Since the patients were young it was decided to reattach the fragments with screws. The heads of the screws were embedded to the level of the surface of the cartilage. Following surgery emphasis was placed on movement without weight-bearing. When the screws were removed three months later, the cartilage fragment appeared to be healthy and healed and the heads of the screws had been covered with newly formed cartilage (Fig. 1). In an arthroscopic examination one year after the accident, no difference could be

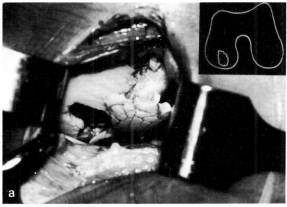

a

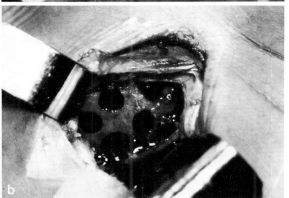

b

Fig. 2. 30 year old ski racer (a). An isolated, 10 cm² shear injury of the medial condyle of the femur. For localization – see sketch (b). Removal of the detached cartilage fragment and pridie forage six weeks after injury

discovered between the formally detached cartilage and normal, healthy, articular cartilage. The line of the fracture was only recognizable as a direct notch.

Although it was generally accepted that fragments of cartilage should be excised [7] our experience to date suggests that a fragment of cartilage which is essentially undamaged should be replaced. It must be of adequate size and the subchondral bone should bleed. Replacement should be limited to children and the younger age group. The nourishment of the reimplanted cartilage is not the main problem, but rather the problem lies in the stability of the new union between the cartilage and the subchondral bone. This will not be as stable as the original fixation but is certainly as good or better than fibrocartilage which would form in such a defect. The one case where the original cartilage had to be removed, a large fragment of regenerated cartilage separated, requiring another arthrotomy two years after the first procedure. The regenerated cartilage appeared softer than the reimplanted cartilage as long as the latter remains healthy. The key is to recognize the shear injury early so that the fragment can be reimplanted before it becomes damaged and while the subchondral bed remains healthy.

References

1. Bandi, W.: Orthopäde **3,** 201 (1974)
2. Benninghoff, A.: Z. Anat. (Lond.) **76,** 43 (1948)
3. Coleman, H. M.: J. Bone Jt. Surg. **30 B,** 1953 (1948)
4. Ganz, R.: H. Unfallheilkunde **110,** 146 (1972)
5. Kennedy, J. C., Wayne Granger, R., Mc Graw, R. W.: J. Bone Jt. Surg. **48 B,** 436 (1966)
6. Morscher, E., Pfeiffer, K.: Vortrag an der 55. Jahresversammlung der Schweiz. Ges. Unfallmed. Berufskr. Interlaken (1966)
7. O'Donoghue, D. H.: Trauma **6,** 469 (1966)
8. Pridie, K. H.: J. Bone Jt. Surg. **37 B,** 350 (1955)
9. Trillat, A., Dejour, H.: Rev. Chir. orthop. **53,** 331 (1967)
10. Wagner, H.: Orthopäde **3,** 208 (1974)

Translation from the German: Isolierte Knorpelabscherungen am Kniegelenk. In: Knorpelschaden am Knie, 4. Reisensburger Workshop zur klinischen Unfallchirurgie, edited by C. Burri and A. Rüter. In: Hefte zur Unfallheilkunde, Vol. 127 (1976). © Springer-Verlag 1976.

Internal Fixation of Osteochondral Fragments

E. H. Kuner and M. Häring

Articular cartilage is an avascular tissue. Nonetheless, there is enough diffusion of molecular contents to maintain an active metabolism. Investigations by Cotta indicate there are two coexisting means of cartilage nutrition [1]. The basal cartilage layer is nourished through the subchondral bone, while the articular surface is nourished by diffusion of synovial fluid. Thus it would appear that there is a junction between the two sources of nutrition within the cartilage layer similar to the junction in the aorta between the intima and media. This junction is particularly susceptible to degenerative change and is more vulnerable to a traumatic displacement. Poorly nourished articular cartilage can no longer fulfill its function, namely protection of the underlying bone by absorption of compressive forces. This results in irreversible damage to the cartilage layer and considerable loss of function in the affected joint.

Careful, anatomically precise, rigid fixation of a displaced intraarticular osteochondral fragment with a normal surface can be achieved. Prerequisites are that the fragment itself is not severely damaged and that the underlying subchondral bone is not excessively thick. Stable fixation allowing early motion must be possible. Restriction of weight-bearing for about 12–16 weeks is necessary.

Goertler [3] has called attention to the value of motion for normal cartilage metabolism. He was able to prove that different positions have a significant influence on the circulation within the capsule. When the knee is flexed, synovial vessels are filled and with the high filtration pressure more molecular constituents can extravasate into the joint cavity. At the same time there are higher osmotic pressures in the vessels of the venous side promoting reabsorption. When the knee is extended, however, and there is insufficient movement these synovial villi collapse and the vessels contract. In this position a large portion of the arterial blood is not utilized. Nourishment of the basal cartilage is deficient. Since the fragments being replaced are autologous, the question of rejection on an immunobiologic basis does not arise.

Three cases will be presented to illustrate our technique when confronted with an acute, displaced, osteochondral fracture.

Case 1:
A 33-year-old woman was kicked on her right knee by a horse. This resulted in a osteochondral fracture of the lateral femoral condyle. The fragment was located in the weight-

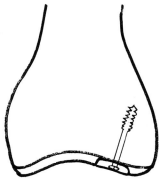

Fig. 1. The displaced osteochondral fragment must be fitted precisely. The head of the screw must be countersunk

bearing zone and was approximately the size of a 25 cent piece. It was obviously displaced. The patient was referred to us fifteen days after the accident and explored the following day. With the knee flexed the fragment could be fitted precisely. It was first fixed with two K-wires and then stabilized by two small cancellous screws. Active movement was begun on the 2nd postoperative day and weight-bearing was restricted for twelve weeks. The wound healed by primary intention.

The screws were removed 50 weeks after the injury. At this time a biopsy was taken from the former fragment. The grossly normal hyaline cartilage also appeared normal histologically. Two and a half years following the procedure the patient was free of complaints and physical examination was normal.

Case 2:
A 16-year-old girl fell from a motorbicycle, landing in such a way as to sustain a displaced osteochondral fracture of the lateral femoral condyle. This was explored four hours following the accident and replaced. The screws were removed 12 weeks later and biopsy again showed healthy hyaline articular cartilage. Macroscopically, the fragment had healed precisely. At follow-up one and a half years later the patient was symptom free and had no abnormal physical findings.

Case 3:
A 33-year-old woman fell backward down a hill sustaining a twist and a direct blow to the left knee. She was seen one day following the injury with a displaced osteochondral fracture of the lateral femoral condyle. This was fixed on the second day following the injury with screws. Fixation was sufficiently stable to allow early active motion. Screws were removed at 17 weeks and at that time a biopsy was taken showing normal hyaline cartilage in the completely healed fragment. At follow-up one and one half years later she was symptom free with normal function.

Three cases of osteochondral fracture of the lateral femoral condyle have been presented. Prompt fixation of these fragments by means of screws provided sufficient stability that the knee could withstand early active motion. This resulted in restoration of a normal articular surface which was confirmed by histological examination at the time of screw removal and by clinical and radiological follow-up one and half to two and a half years later.

References

1. Cotta, H.: Zur Physiologie der Gelenke. Langenbecks Arch. Chir. **316,** 391 (1966)
2. Dustmann, H. O., W. Puhl: Die Reaktion des Gelenkknorpels nach chondralen und osteochondralen Verletzungen. Langenbecks Arch. Chir. 65–66, Forum 1973

3. Goertler, K.: Cavitäre und aniologische Besonderheiten des Kniegelenkes und deren Bedeutung für die Aussagekraft diagnostischer Kapselausschneidungen. Verh. dtsch. Ges. Path. 43. Tagg. 85 (1959)
4. Jonasch, E.: Das Kniegelenk. Berlin: W. de Gruyter, 1964
5. Otte, P.: Biologie des Gelenkknorpels im Hinblick auf die Transplantation. Z. Orthop. **110,** 677 (1972)

Translation from the German: Zur Verschraubung intraarticulärer Knorpel-Knochen-fragmente am Kniegelenk. In: Knorpelschaden am Knie, 4. Reisensburger Workshop zur klinischen Unfallchirurgie, edited by C. Burri and A. Rüter. In: Hefte zur Unfallheil-kunde, Vol. 127 (1976). © Springer-Verlag 1976.

An Experimental Basis for Cartilage Transplantation

W. Hesse and I. Hesse

Introduction

Since the beginning of the 20th century, articular cartilage transplantation has become of increasing interest to both scientists and clinicians. Homologous transplantation of entire human knee joints was reported by Lexer in 1908. At first, good functional results were obtained but the transplanted joints went on to show progressive deformation with osteophytes and erosions of the hyaline articular cartilage. The problems of transplantation of partial or entire joints were shown by the experiments of Herndon and Chase [11]. They used autologous as well as both fresh and frozen homologous bone cartilage transplants in dogs. After varying intervals of time both types of transplants succumbed to necrosis.

Experimental and clinical cartilage transplants have been reported by a number of authors. Among them Campbell [1], Cech [2], De Palma et al. [3], Fiala and Herout [8], Pap and Krompecher [16], Rahmanzadeh [17], Hellinger et al. [10], Hjertquist and Lemperg [12], Sengupta [19], Störig [20], and Wagner [21]. In part excellent results were obtained but transplantation has not become a standard method for the treatment of cartilage damage. There are various reasons for this, but all hinge on one central problem: maintaining the viability of transplanted hyaline cartilage. A transplant can only be regarded as successful if the survival of the hyaline cartilage is assured, and the tissue meets the functional demands. In general, autologous cartilage transplantation completely satifies these prerequisites. However, since there is a limited supply of tissue for autologous transplantation, its use is quite restricted. Fresh homologous transplantation meets with skepticism since the immunologic question is not sufficiently clarified. Furthermore, there are organizational and financial difficulties associated with the use of preserved homologous translants; these can be reduced by the use of a tissue bank. Preservation however, signifies a risk of reduction in viability. To date, no method of preservation is known which maintains the viability of the majority of chondrocytes. It is then understandable that the majority of cases reported in the literature describe necrosis and disintegration of preserved homologous transplants. In both autologous and homologous transplants, the larger the size the smaller the chance for success; this would appear to be dependent on nutritional factors. Thus the most important factors on which cartilage transplantation depends are: viability, type of transplant, preservation, immunology, and nutrition. Any research must take these factors into account. In order to evaluate the characteristics and the function of transplanted articular cartilage, reliable methods should be used whenever possible. These include autoradiography, biochemistry, transmission electron microscopy, and scanning electron microscopy. Evaluation of the transplants should be based on the comparison of healthy and pathologically altered cartilage, as well as the results of the variable surgical methods otherwise available.

Experimental Model

Our experiments were performed on 150 rabbits. We purposely chose a simple model for our experiments. A bone-cartilage defect 3.4 mm in diameter and 3.5 mm in depth was made on the medial femoral condyle of the right knee. The defect was covered with either autologous or preserved homologous bone cartilage transplants or autologous spongiosa. Transplants were preserved for ten days in physiologic saline solution at $+4°C$, in a cyalite[1] solution, and in liquid nitrogen according to Wagner's method. After 2, 4, 6, 12, 18, and 24 months five animals in each group were killed for a total of 25 animals. Examination of the tissue was then carried out by light microscopy, electron microscopy and autoradiography.

X-ray Findings

During the entire two-year period of the experiments, X-ray of the autologous and homologous transplants preserved in liquid nitrogen showed no arthritic changes. Joint space was not narrowed nor were there any irregularities in the joint contour. The transplant showed bony union and it was indistinguishable

---

[1] A mercurial antiseptic (sodium-2-ethylmecurithiobenzoxazole-5-carboxylate).

from the surrounding tissue at the transplant site. Neither radiolucency from osteolysis nor increased radiodensity from sclerosis could be identified.

Microscopic Findings

Grossly good results were found in autologous and homologous transplants preserved in liquid nitrogen. After an examination period of 12 to 24 months one could barely identify the transplant site. The defect was barely recognizable. The transplants preserved in physiologic saline or cyalite or the defects which had been untreated or treated with autologous spongiosa showed poor results; there was evidence of progressive joint degeneration.

Short-term Results

Both the autologous transplants and the homologous transplants preserved in liquid nitrogen showed the same layer depths and the same three-layer form as the surrounding transplant site after 2 and 4 months. The cells in the transplant showed no specific alterations to distinguish them from normal cartilage cells (Fig. 1).

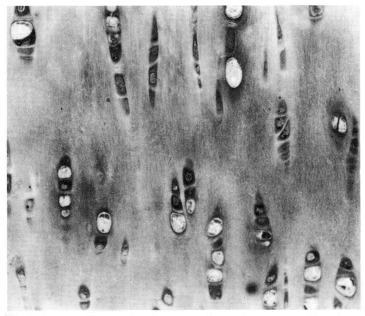

Fig. 1. Intermediate and radiate zone of an autologous cartilage transplant 2 months after transplantation (toluidine blue, 390 ×)

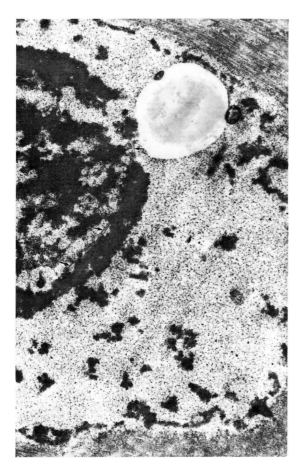

Fig. 2. Section of a dying chon-
droblast 2 months after an autologous transplantation. Vestiges
of the inner and outer nuclear
membrane and fragments of the
plasma membrane can still be
perceived (185 000 ×)

However, in addition to the normal cartilage cells there were many dead and degenerating cells which could be identified by electron microscopy. These were associated with masses of electron dense material in which no cell structure could be identified. It is interesting that a seam of fine fibrils outlines this area just as in normal cartilage cells, but then gradually changes over to coarser fibrils (Fig. 2). At this time the interarticular fissure is bridged by bone. In the cartilaginous areas on the other hand, nonspecific granulation tissue separates the transplant from its bed. Specific mononuclear infiltrates were not observed in either the autologous or homologous transplants. Near the interarticular space at the transplant site numerous clusters of cartilaginous cells were apparent. The overall number of cells in such clusters is definitely not as large as in the clusters which accompany arthrosis. Light microscopy of both autologous and homologous transplants preserved in liquid nitrogen showed viability of cartilage cells 2 months after the transplantation. The layer depths of the transplant, the distribution of the cells, and the appearance of the intercellular matrix were similar to those of normal articular cartilage. The basal calcareous zone remained unchanged. Neither vascular breakdown nor mononuclear cell infiltration was observed. On the other hand electron microscopy revealed many dead and degenerating cells. We, therefore, conclude that both autologous and homologous transplants are no longer fully viable at this point but show changes which must be regarded as regressive. These results contradict those of numerous other authors such as Campbell [1], De Palma [3], Fiala and Herout [8], Pap and Krompecher [16], Störig [20], who, after performing similar experiments, reported the complete survival of the autologous cartilage transplants. One must remember that their statements were based only on light microscopy. De Palma et al. [4] had found that despite the healthy appearance of cartilage under light microscopy, autoradiography had demonstrated impaired concentration of S-35 in their transplants. Herndon and Chase [11] found severe necrosis and degeneration of larger autologous and homologous total joint transplants; these changes were recognizable by light microscopy. Light microscopic assessment of cartilage is only adequate to identify extreme alterations in the cartilage cells. In our experiments the regressive changes were maximal after 2 to 4 months. In autologous transplants less than one-half of all cells survived but in homologous transplants preserved in liquid nitrogen, only a few chondroblasts survived. All cells were necrotic in the homologous transplants preserved by the other methods.

What are the causes for these regressive alterations?

Since in the case of autologous transplantation the rate of necrosis is very high and in the case of homologous transplants no plasma cells, lymphocytes or macrophages were identified, it is unlikely that these are due to immunologic factors. It is our opinion that temporarily inadequate nutrition is responsible for the regressive phase. In contrast to the transplantation bed, the transplanted cells are temporarily separated from the subchondral bone. This then significantly inhibits the nutritional supply to the transplants leading to the death of numerous cells. According to Otte [15], nutrients can only be supplied from the synovium via the interarticular space because of the impermeability of the basal calcareous zone. Fassbender [7] believes that the survival of chondrocytes is completely dependent on the diffusion of proteins and electrolytes from the intraarticular space. These views contrast with our results since in our experimental model the nutritional supply from the spongiosa is the same for both the transplant and the remaining articular cartilage. Nevertheless, the cartilage about the transplantation bed remains viable, while the transplanted cells exhibit extensive cell death. The osseous bed, therefore, must play an important role in the nutrition of the articular cartilage. Morphologically, there is no proof that the basal calcareous zone represents an impermeable barrier to the exchange of substances. The different rate of necrosis for autologous transplants in comparison to the preserved homologous transplants can be explained by the loss of viability incurred during preservation. It is noteworthy that preservation in liquid nitrogen appears to be the only method of preservation in which at least some of the cartilage cells survived.

Midterm Results

At 6 to 12 months a new morphologic pattern presents itself in all cases of autologous transplants and in a majority of homologous transplants preserved in
liquid nitrogen. The number of cells increases but the overall thickness of the
layer decreases. The upper zone of the transplant is occupied by thin, spindle-
shaped cells surrounded by intercellular matrix which is fibrillar by light microscopy. In the lower zone larger cells surrounded by a homogeneously stained
halo are present. A wider and more cellular basal calcareous zone is present
deep to this. With the transmission electron microscope the cells of the upper
zone are identifiable as fibroblasts. Often they are closely packed together, have
non-branching cell processes, and few micropinocytotic vesicles. Coarse fibrils
with the typical periodicity of collagen intimately enveloped the fibroblasts
(Fig. 3). The cells in the lower layer of the transplant cartilage have an extremely
well-developed rough endoplasmic reticulum, numerous vesicles, and prominent
sacs in the Golgi apparatus. In addition, one can identify numerous mitochondria, intracytoplasmic filaments, membrane-bound vesicles with the features of
lysosomes and glycogen particles (Fig. 4). The micropinocytotic vesicles are the
most striking and have two morphologic patterns. Some have a smooth wall
while others which usually are larger, are delineated by a membrane exhibiting
small spikes. The appearance of these micropinocytotic vesicles corresponds to
the so-called "coated vesicles." The 6 to 12 month phase both in autologous and
in the majority of homologous transplants preserved in liquid nitrogen is charac-

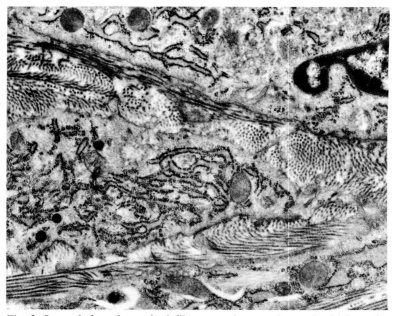

Fig. 3. Several densely packed fibrocytes from a 6-month-old homologous transplant
preserved in liquid nitrogen (18,000 ×)

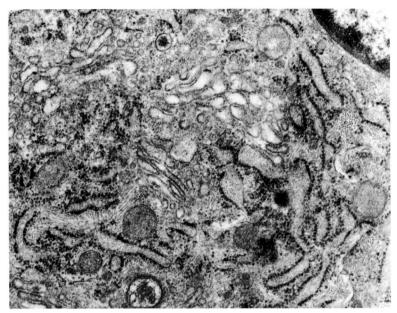

Fig. 4. Section of a cell from the lower zone of an autologous transplant 6 months after transplantation. Noteworthy are the distinctly coarse endoplasmic reticulum, the extended Golgi complex and the numerous mitochondria (41,000 ×)

terized by reparative processes. There are two recognizable cell patterns; the upper layer abounds in fibroblasts and the lower layer is denoted by chondroblasts which at the ultrastructural level are considered extremely active. The autoradiographic studies of Revel and Hay [18] have shown that the synthesis of collagen and of proteoglycans occurs first in the rough endoplasmic reticulum and later in the Golgi apparatus.

Mitochondria supply the energy for these processes. Therefore, in the case of chondrocytes, increased rough endoplasmic reticulum, enlarged Golgi apparatus, and a large number of mitochondria are indicative of intensified collagen and proteoglycan synthesis.

Micropinocytotic vesicles play a role in resorption. The micropinocytotic vesicles whose membrane shows small spikes, the so-called "coated vesicles", are associated with resorption of protein. On the basis of the present experiments, it is impossible to know whether these active chondrocytes are surviving transplanted chondrocytes, or whether they are transformed fibroblasts arising from the basal zone of the transplant bed.

Longterm Results

In the final 12 to 24 months after transplantation, the appearance of autologous and homologous transplants preserved in liquid nitrogen becomes increasingly similar. The more superficial layer of the transplant is still thinned but the

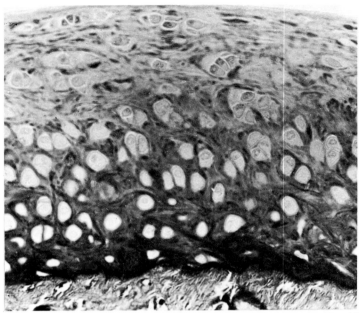

Fig. 5. Appearance of a homologous transplant preserved in liquid nitrogen 18 months after the transplantation (PAS stain, 390 ×)

appearance of the transplant resembles more and more hyaline articular cartilage. Large areas of the transplants show cells of varying shapes and size which are usually clustered in groups. In the lower zones larger, rounded, and usually single cells are found which resemble normal chondrocytes (Fig. 5). By autoradiography the transplanted cells show a normal aggregation of S-35 in all zones. Electron microscopy shows that the oval cells have irregular, extensively branched long cellular processes. The presence of micropinocytotic vesicles, a well-developed endoplasmic reticulum, densely invested with ribosomes and lysosomelike bodies all indicate that these are metabolically active cells. Collagen fibrils of varying thickness surround these cells. In addition masses of a fine filamentous tangle can be seen (Fig. 6). The variable appearance of the intercellular matrix reflects the variable synthetic activity of the cells. A second cell type is characterized by larger, round cells. These have short cellular processes uniformly distributed over the cell surface. Micropinocytotic vesicles are less frequent. Rough endoplasmic reticulum is also reduced. Usually intracytoplasmic filaments and clusters of glycogen particles are seen in these cells. Seams of fine collagenous fibrils surround some of these cells. The appearance is that of normal chondrocytes from hyaline cartilage.

Scanning electron microscopy of autologous and homologous transplants preserved in liquid nitrogen shows that after 12 to 24 months the appearance of the transplant is uniform. Funicular protrusions bordered by groovelike depresions are characteristic features. These occur in parallel groups, as well as in groups that intersect or converge on one another. They are not all at one level

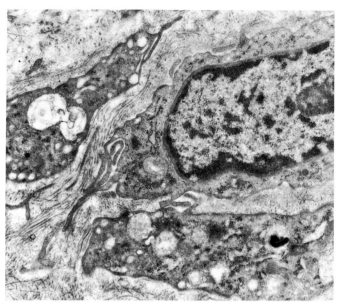

Fig. 6. Cells gathered together in groups in the upper zone of a 12-month-old autologous transplant. The appearance of the surrounding intercellular substance varies (16,800 X)

but cross both above and below one another. Their surface has a fibrillary texture which surrounds them in a netlike fashion. In many areas there is a leveling of the groovelike depressions, and the cordlike fibrillar structures are no longer distinctly discernible and the surface is more homogeneous (Fig. 7). In some cases, in particular at the center of the transplant, a substantial similarity to the original articular cartilage can be identified. The superficial structure of autologous and of homologous transplant preserved in liquid nitrogen is altered when compared to the normal articular cartilage. However, the morphological picture does not suggest destruction. On the contrary, the scanning electron-microscopic findings suggest repair of the cartilage surface. This can be illustrated by considering comparable situations. A clear-cut differentiation can be made from arthrotic cartilage which is characterized by severe destruction at the surface. Tears, pits, defects, fibrillar shreds exhibiting plaquelike disintegration are typical for arthrotic articular cartilage. Destructive processes are predominant in the cases of homologous transplants preserved in physiologic saline at 4°C or preserved in cyalite solution. With increasing matrix loss the fibrils are undermined, then exposed, and then they break off producing extensive cavitation (Fig. 8).

What happens when a cartilage bone defect the size of our transplant is left to heal by itself and not covered by a transplant? Plaquelike and tattered disintegration of the newly formed fibrillar masses and the so-called flow formations reveal an unsuccessful attempt to repair the cartilage surface. Large empty spaces are often covered by only a few fibers which are disconnected and show spikelike projections. The fissure between the transplant and the recipient bid is

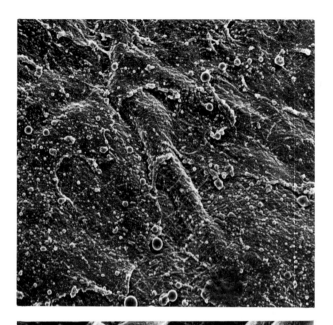

Fig. 7. Surface of an auto-logous transplant 18 months after transplan-tation. On the homoge-nous surface, funicular fibrillar traits appear only sporadically (3000 ×)

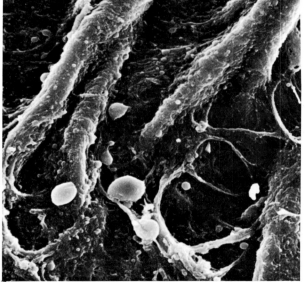

Fig. 8. Surface of a homol-ogous transplant preserv-ed in a physiologic saline solution. The exposed fibers and extensive cavity formations are charac-teristic (6000 ×)

regarded as a microdefect; it represents a discontinuity of the basal calcareous zone. The important question is whether a spanning with cartilage is possible. Otte [15] writes that although it can result in fusion of the subchondral bony layer with the analogous host tissue, it cannot result in fusion of the cartilage. The area of the fissure in our experiments exhibited a variable appearance. In many areas it is occupied by densely packed, ropelike, and fibrillar structures. Simultaneously broad foliaceous structures cover this fissure. Their ends are sometimes thinly cylindric and at other times down apart in cuspidate fashion

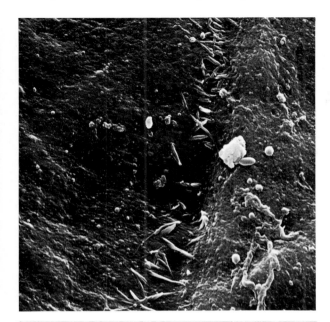

Fig. 9. Fissure area spanned by structures which are terracelike, piled upon each other, broad, and foliaceous, the so-called flow formations (120 ×)

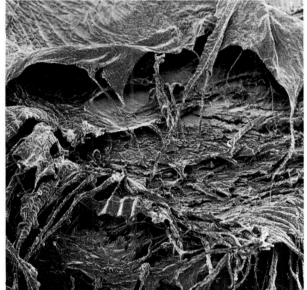

Fig. 10. Location where the original fissure area is completely spanned (6000 ×)

(Fig. 9). At numerous locations a complete spanning of the fissure develops showing several intermediate stages (Fig. 10).

According to the investigations carried out by Ghadially et al. [9] on cartilage defects, the so-called cartilage flow is not merely a phenomenon which leads to a rounding-off of the defective crests, but also plays a significant role in filling the defect. Under certain conditions the so-called flow formation is capable of affecting a fusion of the cartilage. This contradicts Otte's [15] statement that a fusion of the cartilage is basically not possible.

It seems possible that in addition to the above-mentioned prerequisites, it is necessary that deep in the fissure the granulation tissue transforms itself into cartilaginous tissue. All autologous and homologous bone cartilage transplants initially passed through a regressive phase of varying intensity. This fact could be of significant importance within the framework of postoperative treatment. For this reason it is necessary to offer the joint temporary rest from use. This is followed by a regeneration phase in the case of autologous and homologous transplants preserved in liquid nitrogen. Although even after 2 years no morphologically normal articular cartilage with the original layer depths and typical three-layer formation has developed, nevertheless, the tissue exists which substantially consists of hyaline chondrocytes, and which under the scanning electron microscope exhibits an ordered and regular superficial structure. This, we consider a process of repair of the articular cartilage. Our long-term results, however, cannot be put on a par with those of Herndon and Chase [11] who report a corrosion of the cartilage transplants. On the contrary, our positive long-term results resemble those of Pap and Krompecher [16]. However, based on electron microscopy, we cannot share the opinion that autologous transplants survive without any indication of necrosis.

Immunology

In agreement with what has been reported in the literature homologous cartilage transplants furnish no evidence of immunologic reaction. The question arises as to whether articular cartilage occupies a special immunologic position. In 1974 Langer, Gross, and Elves reported on this. They were able to prove that only isolated chondrocytes possessed antigenic characteristics. Intact articular cartilage and chondrocytes not surrounded by matrix do not stimulate immunologic reactions. From these results one concludes that immunologic problems in homologous cartilage transplantations can only be of secondary importance. This, therefore, equates autologous and fresh homologous cartilage transplants with regards to the usefulness of the transplantation.

Surgical Alternatives

The reimplantation of traumatically dislodged bone cartilage fragments or of dissected fragments in osteochondritis dissecans is routinely performed in our clinic. One must, however, clearly understand that this cartilaginous tissue always exhibits cellular necrosis by transmission electron microscopy and alterations of the superficial structure under scanning electron microscopy. Even in cases of bone cartilage fragments which appear macroscopically sound, we were always able to observe tattered and flaplike structures.

Summary

On the whole, autologous cartilage transplantation still offers the best chance for repair of cartilage defects. Under certain conditions homologous cartilage transplants preserved in liquid nitrogen also present a good chance for success. Thus cartilage transplantation has a fundamental therapeutic potential in the sense of a temporally limited repair of a cartilage defect which permits the maintenance of the joint's function.

References

1. Campbell, C. J.: Homotransplantation of a half or whole joint Clin. Orthop. Rel. Res. **87,** 146 (1972)
2. Cech, O.: Rekonstruktion des Hüftgelenkes mit autologer Knorpelkappe Z. Orthop. **110,** 714 (1972)
3. De Palma, A. F., Sawyer, B., Hoffmann, J. D.: Fate of osteochondral grafts. Clin. Orthop. **22,** 217 (1962)
4. De Palma, A. F., Tsaltas, T. T., Maurer, G. G.: Viability of osteochondral grafts as determined by uptake of S. 35. J. Bone Jt. Surg. **45 A,** 1565 (1963)
5. Ehalt, W.: Gelenkknorpelplastik. Langenbecks Arch. Chir. **299,** 768 (1962)
6. Elves, M.: A study of the transplantation antigens on chondrocytes from articular cartilage. J. Bone Jt. Surg. **56 B,** 178 (1974)
7. Fassbender, H. G.: Pathologie rheumatischer Erkrankungen. Berlin–Heidelberg–New York: Springer 1975
8. Fiala, O., Herout, V.: Experimentelle homologe Transplantation von Gelenkteilen und ganzer Gelenke. Z. Orthop. **110,** 691 (1972)
9. Ghadially, F. N., Ailsby, R. L., Oryschak, A. F.: Scanning electron microscopy of superficial defects in articular cartilage. Ann. rheum. Dis. **33,** 327 (1974)
10. Hellinger, J., Siegling, C. W., Brauckhoff, K. F., Schramm, G.: Vitale autologe und homologe Halbgelenkstransplantation im Tierexperiment. Beitr. Orthop. **21,** 617 (1974)
11. Herndon, C. H., Chase, S. W.: Experimental studies in transplantation of whole joints. J. Bone Jt. Surg. **34 A,** 564 (1952)
12. Hjertquist, S. O., Lemperg, R.: Long term observations in the articular cartilage and autologous costal cartilage transplanted to osteochondral defects on the femoral head. Calcif. Tiss. Res. **9,** 226 (1972)
13. Langer, F., Gross, A. E.: Immunogenicity of allograft articular cartilage. J. Bone Jt. Surg. **56 A,** 297 (1974)
14. Lexer, E.: Substitution of whole or half joints from freshly amputated extremities by free plastic operation. Surg. Gynec. Obstet. **6,** 601 (1908)
15. Otte, P.: Die Verpflanzung von Gelenkknorpeln. Z. Orthop. **110,** 677 (1972)
16. Pap, K., Krompecher, S.: Arthroplasty of the knee, experimental and clinical experiences. J. Bone Jt. Surg. **43 A,** 523 (1961)
17. Rahmanzadeh, R.: Die Problematik des osteocartilaginären Gewebsersatzes. Mschr. Unfallheilk. **75,** 248 (1972)
18. Revel, J. P., Hay, E. D.: An autoradiographic and electron microscopic study of collagen synthesis in differentiating cartilage. Z. Zellforsch. **61,** 110 (1963)
19. Sengupta, S.: The fate of transplants of articular cartilage in the rabbit. J. Bone Jt. Surg. **56 B,** 167 (1974)

20. Störig, E.: Knorpeltransplantation im Tierexperiment und Erfahrungen über ihre klinische Anwendung. Z. Orthop. **110,** 685 (1972)
21. Wagner, H.: Möglichkeiten und klinische Erfahrungen mit der Knorpeltransplantation. Z. Orthop. **110,** 708 (1972)

This work was carried out with support from the Deutsche Forschungsgemeinschaft. We would like to thank Professor, Dr. Reale, Head of the Institute for Electron Microscopy of the Medizinische Hochschule, Hannover for his continued assistance.

Translation from the German: Experimentelle Grundlagen der Knorpeltransplantation. In: Knorpelschaden am Knie, 4. Reisensburger Workshop zur klinischen Unfallchirurgie, edited by C. Burri and A. Rüter. In: Hefte zur Unfallheilkunde, Vol. 127 (1976). © Springer-Verlag 1976.

Osteochondrosis Dissecans

W. Müller

The clinical picture of osteochondritis dissecans of the knee is typical and usually follows a predictable course, but the etiology remains unclear. Although inflammatory changes are rarely seen, the English and French literature continue to call this an osteochondritis dissecans. In the German literature the concept of osteochondrosis dissecans has appeared but even this terminology does not help clarify the cause. The two most popular etiologic theories are hereditary predisposition or trauma.

Osteochondral alterations are characteristically present on convex articular surfaces, not only in the knee joint, but e.g., over the capitellum of the humerus or the metatarsal head. This suggests that circulatory problems are important for those articular surfaces which protrude into a joint. Either the blood supply is not capable of nourishing all epiphyseal parts, or single or repetitive trauma results in a subchondral ischemia with an area of osteochondral necrosis. It is quite possible that microfractures of the fine cancellous bone in the sense of a fatigue fracture are present. In an exposed convex surface a pseudarthrosis would lead to a permanent circulatory block to the fragment and spontaneous dissection. Injuries in the articular cartilage would then be the result of differences in elasticity of the unstable osseous substructure in the area beneath the affected articular cartilage.

Diagnosis of Osteochondritis

In younger patients during the growing years the clinical picture is associated with vague knee pain, sporadic effusion with swelling usually secondary to stress. Locking by a extruded fragment occurs at an older age. In addition to a complete physical examination of the knee appropriate X-rays are essential (Fig. 1). In addition to the routine AP and lateral X-rays, a 90° X-ray as described by Frick and a tangential view of the patella should be included. Occasionally tomograms are helpful. In rare cases arthroscopy or arthrotomy is needed to confirm the diagnosis.

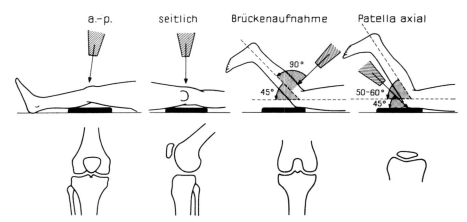

Fig. 1. Important standard X-rays of the knee joint in the case of osteochondrosis dissecans

Differential Diagnosis

A fresh impression fracture of the condyle must be excluded as well as an osteochondral fracture after patellar dislocation. The osteocartilaginous fragment usually exhibits multiple infractions. Finally one should not forget direct trauma to the articular cartilage by contusion or compression of a meniscus in a hyperextended knee (Fig. 2). A pedunculated tear of the posterior horn of the medial meniscus with chronic interposition can produce a large cartilaginous ulcer on the medial condyle. In the older age group, avascular osteonecrosis of the femoral condyle must be considered. This condition may not be radiologically evident for several months but is frequently visible in a bone scan.

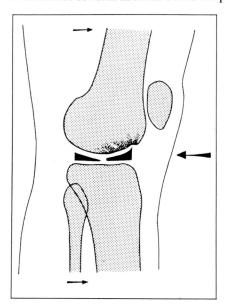

Fig. 2. An impression with cartilage damage on the femoral condyle caused by hyperextension

Treatment of Osteochondrosis Dissecans (O.D.)

Conservative Treatment

Conservative or nonoperative treatment predisposes a tendency toward spontaneous healing in early cases. It can be advocated when osteochondrosis is diagnosed as an incidental finding in children. The following prerequisites exist — no complaints, the focus must be small and largely outside the stress zone, and finally the sclerotic zone bordering the area of the dissected fragment must be narrow. Often these radiological changes may resemble irregularities in growth of the condyle.

Surgical Treatment

In most cases surgery is the treatment of choice. The selection of the surgical procedure will depend on the area of involvement, the state of the articular cartilage over the fragment, the underlying bed, possible dissection, and any associated deformity such as genu varum.

If the focus is located in an exposed weight-bearing area and the articular cartilage is well preserved, forage and perforation of the sclerotic bone with a cancellous graft is possible. In the case of a demarcated cartilage border or a frank loose body, the subchondral bone can be curetted and drilled from the articular surface and the fragment replaced and internally fixed. In the case of a large articular defect where there is no fragment that can be replaced, because it has fragmented or macerated, then an osteochondral transplant is indicated. In the presence of a large area of osteochondritis in the weight-bearing area and an associated genu varum, then a valgus, high tibial osteotomy is the procedure of choice. Each of these possibilities will be considered in detail.

1. Focus in the Weight-bearing Area with Articular Surface Preserved

Open Epiphyseal Plate: The synovial membrane is carefully swept back from the junction of the articular cartilage toward the insertion of the collateral ligament. A window is made in the femoral condyle and through this window the focus of osteochondrosis is packed with cancellous bone (Fig. 3).

Closed Epiphyseal Plate: The window in the femoral condyle can be made much more proximally and in an extraarticular position above the origin of the medial collateral ligament (Fig. 4).

2. Osteochondral Flap or Loose Body

If the articular surface is clearly demarcated or a flap or loose body is present, the sclerotic zone is approached from the articular surface and curetted. The

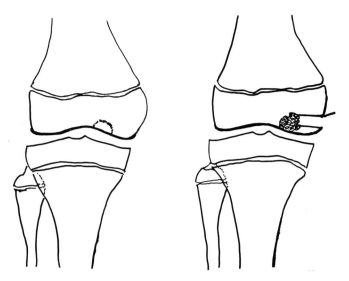

Fig. 3. Technique for underlining with spongiosa in the case of open epiphyseal cartilage

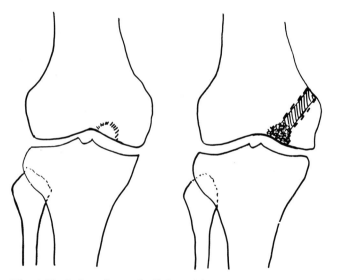

Fig. 4. Technique for underlining with spongiosa in the case of closed epiphyseal cartilage

dissected fragment is then fixed with a screw. To date we have not used Smillie pins. Screw head must be well countersunk.

The reimplantation is confirmed radiologically. The screws are removed as early as six to eight weeks postoperatively prior to full weight-bearing (Fig. 5). The advantage of screws is the compression force for a stable reimplantation.

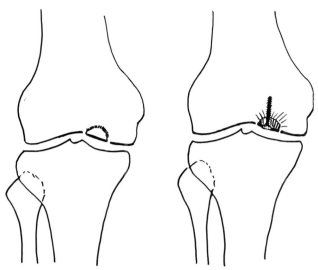

Fig. 5. Technique for freshening the bearing of a dissected fragment by replantation of the dissected fragment and fixation with screws

3. No Frank Dissected Fragment But Severe Cartilage Softening or Multiple Loose Fragments

Should no actual single fragment be present, if there is diffuse softening of the articular surface or even multiple loose bodies, then transplant of articular cartilage is indicated. This may be autologous or homologus. The subject has been discussed extensively by Wagner (Fig. 6).

When the separated fragment is small and not located in an exposed weight-bearing zone, the underlying cancellous bone may simply be curetted with no

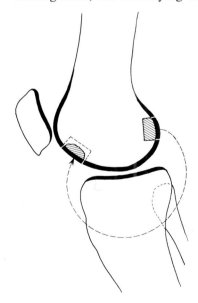

Fig. 6. Implantation of an autotransplant

need to reconstruct the cartilaginous surface. Arthroscopically such a defect can appear to be quite sound 12 weeks following curettage and show a good synovial membrane and a cartilaginous appearance.

A young patient had had two previous operative procedures at other centers for a large osteochondrotic focus on the *lateral* femoral condyle. We removed the remaining fragments and underlying fibrous tissue. The patient had a genu varum so osteotomy was not considered. Fresh, bleeding, cancellous bone was exposed throughout the affected condyle. The knee was then treated by motion without weight-bearing for four months. There was marked improvement and resolution of the chronic effusion. X-ray three years postoperatively showed preservation of the contour of the femoral condyle in this 17-year-old boy. This as well as the previous example indicates that curettage of the base of the defect can be justified in certain cases (Fig. 7).

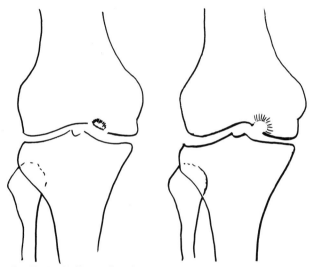

Fig. 7. Technique of a simple removal of the focus and freshening of vital spongiosa if a small focus is located outside of the stress zone

4. Large Defect in Weight-bearing Area with Genu Varum

If a large area of osteochondrosis is present in an exposed weight-bearing area on the medial side in association with the genu varum, a valgus osteotomy is indicated. One patient showed repeated effusions until such an osteotomy was done. Since correction of the angular deformity he has been free of effusion and fit for work for five years now (Fig. 8).

Conclusion

Several general considerations concerning the operative technique and post-operative management of osteochondrosis dissecans of the knee joint should be

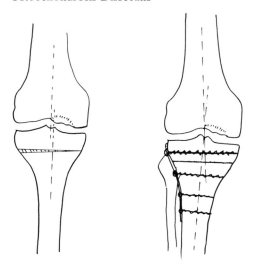

Fig. 8. Technique of a high osteotomy of the tibia in the case of severe osteochondrosis and genu varum

mentioned. Immobilization is undesirable for both healthy and especially damaged articular cartilage. For this reason we encourage immediate post-operative movement. Weight-bearing on the other hand is restricted by means of crutches, until the subchondral bone has united. We use parapatellar approaches and are careful to avoid damage to the sides of the femoral condyles. Care must also be taken to treat the suprapatellar pouch carefully to avoid adhesion and loss of flexion. Special attention must be paid to the details of the operative technique to obtain an optimal result.

References

1. Aichroth, P. M.: Osteochondritis dissecans of the knee. J. Bone Jt. Surg. **51 B,** 181 (1969)
2. Aichroth, P. M.: Osteochondritis dissecans of the knee. J. Bone Jt. Surg. **53 B,** 440 (1971)
3. Bühler, A.: Die hohe Tibiaosteotomie bei Gonarthrose. Diss. Basel 1974
4. Debeyre, J., Gontallier, D.: Traitement par vissage de l'ostéochondrite disséquante de l'extremité inferieure de fémur. Rev. Chir. orthop. **51,** 709 (1965).
5. Duparc, J., Alnot, J. Y.: Ostéonékrose primitive du condyle fémoral interne du sujet agé. Rev. Chir. orthop. **55,** 615 (1969)
6. Helfet, A. J.: The Management of Internal Derangement of the Knee. Philadelphia: Lippincott 1963
7. Ingwerson, O. S., ED.: The Knee Joint. Amsterdam: Excerpta Medica 1974; New York: American Elsevier Publishing
8. Lichtenstein, L.: Diseases of bone and joints. St. Louis: Mosby 1975
9. Mohing, W.: Arthrosis deformans des Kniegelenkes. Berlin—Heidelberg—New York: Springer 1966
10. Morscher, E.: Transplantation von Knochen und Gelenkknorpel. Bulletin schweiz. Akad. med. Wiss. **26,** 287 (1970)
11. Palazzi, A. S.: Autogenous osteocartilaginous grafting for severe lesions of the knee. J. Bone Jt. Surg. **54 B,** 383 (1968)
12. Perreau, M.: Osteochondrite du cotyle fémoral radiologiquement silencieuse. Rev. Chir. orthop. **56,** 792 (1970)

13. Smillie, I. S.: Diseases of the Knee Joint. London-Edinburgh: Livingstone 1974
14. Trillat, A., Dejour, H., Bonsquet, G.: Chirurgie du genou. Lyon: Simep 1971
15. Trillat A.: Les ostéochondrites des condyles fémoraux. Rev. Chir. orthop. **57,** 319 (1971)
16. Wagner, H.: Traitement operatoire de l'osteochondrite dissequante cause de l'arthrite déformante du genou. Rev. Chir. orthop. **-0,** 335 (1964)
17. Wagner, H.: Z. Orthop. **98,** 33 (1964)
18. Wagner, H.: Hefte Unfallheilk. **110,** 140 (1972)
19. Wagner, H.: Traumatische Knorpelschädigungen des Kniegelenkes. Orthopäde **3,** 208 (1974)

Translation from the German: Osteochondrosis dissecans (Diagnose und Therapie). In: Knorpelschaden am Knie, 4. Reisensburger Workshop zur klinischen Unfallchirurgie, edited by C. Burri and A. Rüter. In: Hefte zur Unfallheilkunde, Vol. 127 (1976).
© Springer-Verlag 1976.

Retropatellar Cartilage Degeneration: Diagnosis and Outline of Treatment

A. Rüter and C. Burri

Diagnosis, History, and Physical Examination

Retropatellar arthrosis produces painful malfunction of the patellofemoral joint. The pressure of the patella on the femoral condyles is a function of the flexion of the knee joint. With increasing flexion, the amount of extension force necessary for its neutralization increases the pressure across the patellofemoral joint. This

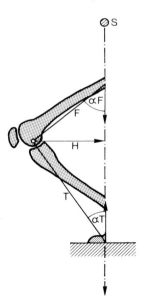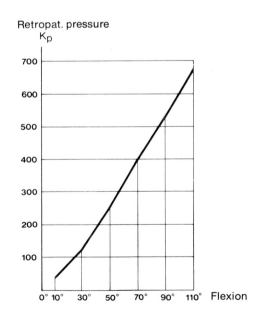

$$H = F \cdot \sin \alpha_F = T \cdot \sin \alpha_T$$

Fig. 1. Geometric functions of the forces active on the knee joint

is in fact a parallelogram of forces. Retropatellar pressure has been calculated by Bandi [1] and tested experimentally (Fig. 1).

Initially pain on hills and stairs may be the only complaint and even in late stages it remains the principle symptom. Descending is usually more painful.

On physical examination, the pain can be provoked by asking the patient to perform a knee-bend on one leg. The patient often refuses as he knows that this will produce severe pain. The examiner can simulate this mechanism by pressure over the patella when the quadriceps are relaxed and request the patient to tighten his quadriceps muscle. The patella is drawn through its facet into axial stress and this leads to the typical pain (Fig. 2). Retropatellar crepitus can often be felt better than heard. The mobility of the patella should also be tested horizontally and vertically. Standard examination of the knee joint, including testing for an effusion, ligament stability, and meniscal integrity are of course also carried out.

Retropatellar cartilage changes do not usually affect the entire surface. The medial and lateral facets must be examined separately. The patella is shifted medially, the medial facet protrudes from the intercondylar fossa, and it can be palpated directly. The lateral facet is also pressed against the condyle (Fig. 3). With lateral displacement of the patella, the lateral facet becomes palpable and the medial facet is compressed (Fig. 4). By determining the point of maximum tenderness, it is possible to differentiate the involvement of the facets.

The examination technique allows one to reach an overall diagnosis of retropatellar arthrosis and to determine the condition of major patellar changes. Further investigation is necessary to clarify the etiology and extent of the complaint. In addition to documenting the nature of the pain, it is important to inquire as to any history of fracture, contusion, injections, or possible infections.

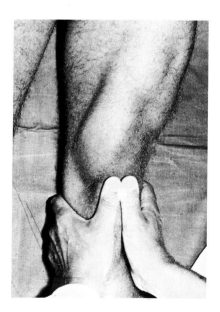

Fig. 2. Examination of the sensitivity of the patellar gliding pathway

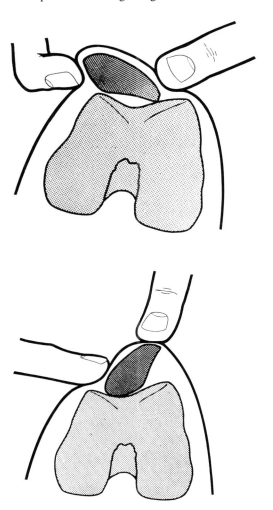

Fig. 3. Palpation of the medial facet

Fig. 4. Palpation of the lateral facet

On radiological examination, AP and lateral views of the knee are necessary. The lateral view may permit some judgement of retropatellar problems. The X-ray can also show the so-called Haglund impression (Fig. 5), a concavity on the deep surface of the patella with a sclerotic face which Haglund [20] describes as a manifestation of contusion to the deep surface. There is no definite agreement concerning its origin or significance.

There are two techniques currently used to assess the relation of the patella to the femur in the lateral view. Blumensaat's [4] method is a lateral view in 30° of flexion (Fig. 6). According to Blumensaat, the patella alta exists in all cases in which the inferior pole is higher than the prolongation of the line between the femoral condyles. The length of the patellar ligament relative to the length of the patella as described by Insall and Salvati [24] is a more reliable method for the diagnosis of patella alta. This should not exceed 1.3.

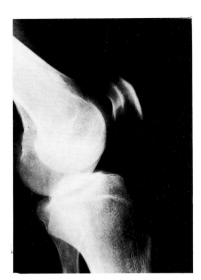

Fig. 5. Haglund's impression

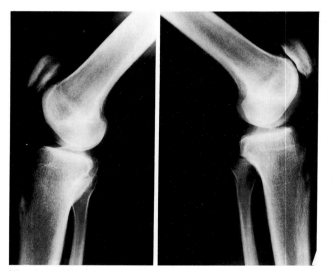

Fig. 6. Patella alta on both sides with retropatellar arthrosis

If there is excessive angulation between the direction of the quadriceps pole and the patellar ligament, there is a tendency for lateral displacement of the patella, accompanied by increased pressure on the lateral facet and loss of medial contact. These axial measurements can only be judged on AP X-rays which extend from at least mid-femur to mid-tibia. The tendency for patellar subluxation can often be demonstrated radiographically when an AP view is taken at the moment of maximal quadriceps contraction. In this X-ray compared to the standard view, both lateral displacement and upward shifting of the patella can be observed (Fig. 7).

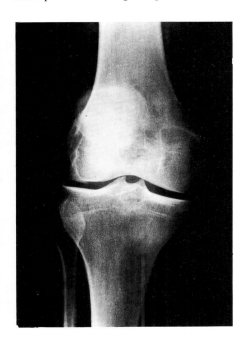

Fig. 7. Anteroposterior X-ray of tightened quadriceps. In the case of chronic subluxation, the patella moves laterally

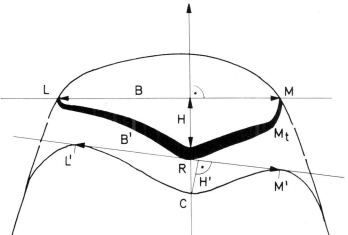

Fig. 8. Lines and angles for the calculation of the indices on the patella and condyles according to Ficat and Bizou

Tangential or skyline views of the patella which permit assessment of the patellofemoral articulation are essential. Ficat and Bizou [10] describe certain indices by which a form of the patellofemoral joint can be classified (Fig. 8). B: H is the depth index of the patella (normal 3.6–4.2) B': H' is the index of the depth of the intercondylar fossa (normal 4.2–6.5); LR:MR is the patellar index which can alternate between 1 and 3; and L-R-M is the angle of one facet to the other (normal 120°–140°). These indices allow classification of patellar

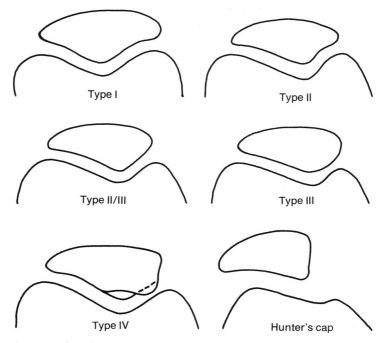

Fig. 9. Various forms of the patella according to Wiberg and Baumgartl

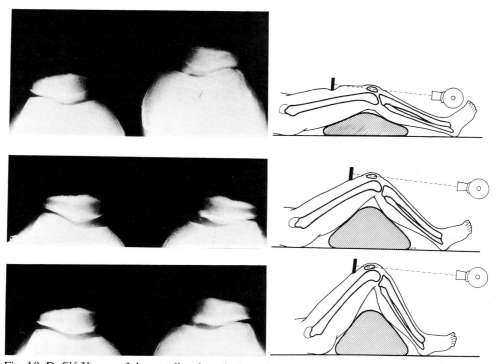

Fig. 10. Defilé X-rays of the patella when the knee joint is flexed at 30°, 60°, and 90°

forms according to Wiberg [37] and Baumgartl [2]. Angles of less than 120° are characteristic of Wiberg's type II and III. These are considered to have a significant association with chondromalacia (Fig. 9). These tangential X-rays may also reveal the ridge on the medial femoral condyle described by Outerbridge [34].

For a straightforward diagnosis the tangential X-rays described are adequate. The degree of flexion at which the X-rays are taken must be determined. The appearance of the patellofemoral joint changes from the distal to the proximal ends so that X-rays taken at different projections cannot be compared. Ficat and Philippe [11] have taken this into consideration and recommended that tangential views be taken at 30°, 60°, and 90° of flexion. At 30° the inferior articulation is seen best, at 60° the midpoint, and at 90° the proximal. These views permit a more precise evaluation of the patellofemoral joint (Fig. 10).

Arthroscopy

This investigation technique is assuming increasing importance in the diagnosis of early cases as well as for the supervision of the course of the disease.

In chondromalacia patellae, as well as establishing the diagnosis of retropatellar degeneration, it should be possible to differentiate the cause more precisely. There are two basic types: Type I – chondromalacia patellae in the presence of an impaired gliding pathway (Fig. 11). Examples are: dysplastic patella–Wiberg II and III, patella alta–Blumensaat, Insall and Salvati; recurrent dislocation of the patella–(case history, AP X-ray with quadriceps contracted) neuromuscular damage caused by quadriceps insufficiency. Type II––chondromalacia patellae in the presence of a disturbed gliding surface. Examples are; posttraumatic (fracture, contusion), primary chondromalacia no pathogenesis apparent and symptomatic forms (as an expression of systemic illness such as osteoporosis, Sudeck's, circulatory disturbance, etc.).

Treatment

Conservative Therapy: There are three basic measures namely, improvement in the mechanics, physical measures, and medication.

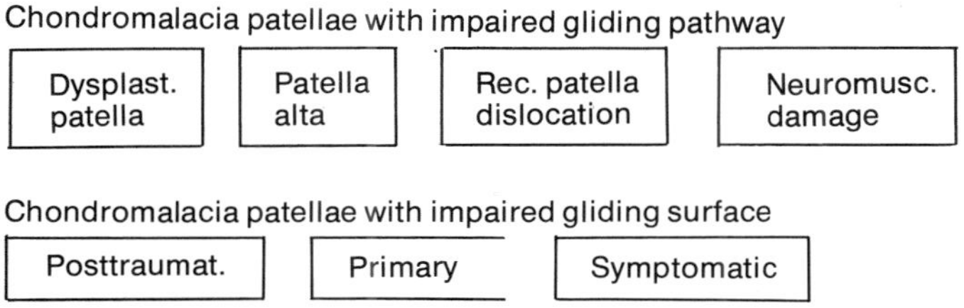

Chondromalacia patellae with impaired gliding pathway

| Dysplast. patella | Patella alta | Rec. patella dislocation | Neuromusc. damage |

Chondromalacia patellae with impaired gliding surface

| Posttraumat. | Primary | Symptomatic |

Fig. 11. Causes of chondromalacia

Retropatellar pressure depends on the degree of flexion of the knee joint but it is also influenced by the body weight. Therefore, weight loss will cause a marked reduction in retropatellar pressure.

Physical Methods: Many local applications including mud, peat, and paraffin have been tried. Cold has been popular recently especially if the knee joint is inflamed. Short-wave diathermy and ultrasound are also used commonly. Some have advocated radiotherapy to eliminate pain receptors, however, patients with recurrent pain after this treatment are resistant to other forms of therapy.

Medication: Analgesics and antiinflammatory medication are indicated in mild cases for symptomatic relief. Other agents containing mixtures of glucose salts and anesthetic agents have been tried. Various cartilage bone extracts are said to support the synthesis of mucopolysaccharides [e.g., 28] but there is little evidence for this.

Surgical Treatment

Procedures to Normalize the Gliding Pathway:

Ninety surgical procedures have been reported. In 1904 Krogius [27] reported the transfer of a strip from the medial to the lateral retinaculum. The Hauser procedure [22] consists of medial displacement of the tibial tubercle and is a common procedure. Goldthwait [16] moved the lateral third of the ligamentum patellae to the medial side. This is especially useful when the epiphyses are still open. Campbell [6] described a strip from the medial retinaculum to the superior patellar pole and sewn back to itself. This medialized the quadriceps. The same effect is achieved by advancing the insertion of the vastus medialis, a method proposed by Green [18] and Madigan [29].

Lateral Facet Compression: Ficat [12] termed the dysbalance where there is excessive pressure on the lateral facet and lack of pressure on the medial "the syndrome of external hypertension." Keyl and Viernstein [26] had described this mechanical problem earlier. They recommended, as Ficat does, splitting the lateral retinaculum. Ficat [13] also resects a strip at least 1 cm wide since in his experience division alone often leads to recurrence.

Patella Alta: Distal displacement of the tibial tubercle (Roux) is the best known procedure for patella alta. Because of the anterior ridge of the tibia in this region, distal displacement leads to posterior patellar displacement. This decreases the lever arm of the extensor apparatus and increases retropatellar pressure. This may aggravate chondromalacia. For this reason Groeneveld [19] suggested a different procedure for these cases. The origin of the patellar

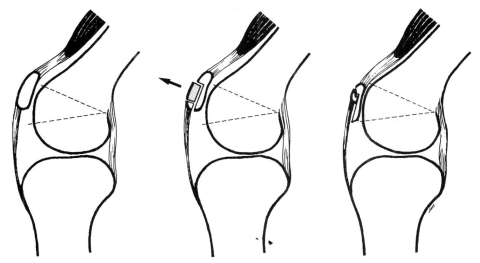

Fig. 12. Operation for patella alta according to Groeneveld

ligament is taken from the inferior pole with a block of bone. A segment is then resected from the anterior surface of the patella and the block is reinserted proximal to its original site. If the block is also shifted posteriorly then forward displacement of the patella is obtained at the same time (Fig. 12).

Operations to Improve the Gliding Surface

Shaving: Simple shaving and removal of coarse and villous cartilaginous pieces appears to be a technically convincing procedure. It is easy, however, to misjudge the residual cartilage quality and gliding ability of the patella.

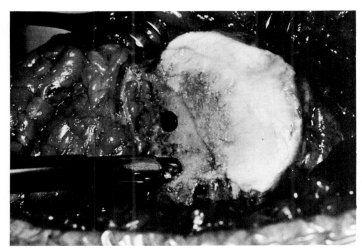

Fig. 13. Drilling according to Pridie

Drilling: Pridie [34] suggested that subchondral sclerosis be pierced by drilling. He felt that cartilage degeneration was caused by nutritional disturbance originating from impaired diffusion from the subchondral layers. Drilling was supposed to pierce the barrier of sclerosis. This procedure is reserved for cases where there is no articular cartilage at all. Granulations of connective tissue from the cancellous bone deep to the sclerotic layer are transformed into fibrocartilage with movement and the cartilage defect is then covered, with a cartilage substitute (Fig. 13).

Interposition: Various materials have been described as interposition grafts of the patellofemoral joint. Such examples were described by Goymann [17] in which he reported a partial tangential patellar resection with interposition of the prepatellar bursa. He recommended as thick a resection as possible so that the retropatellar pressure would also be reduced.

Techniques to Reduce Retropatellar Pressure

Anterior Displacement: The concept of reducing the retropatellar pressure and improving the lever arm of the extensor mechanism was published by Maquet [30]. In his original work he suggested that the patellar tendon be elevated from its insertion at the tuberosity by a corticocancellous graft (Fig. 14). Bandi [1] standardized the surgical procedure so that the tibial tubercle is displaced anteriorly a precise distance (Fig. 15).

Patellectomy: Patellectomy is the most radical method of dealing with this problem. In addition to weakening the joint, the possible influence on the femoral and tibial articulations must be considered. Fürmaier [14] calculated

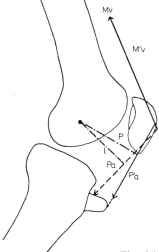

Fig. 14. Operation according to Maquet

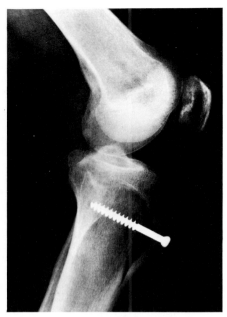

Fig. 15. Operation according to Bandi

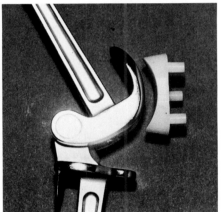

Fig. 16. Münster patella in the case
of a Guepar knee

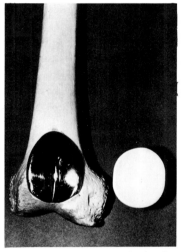

Fig. 17. Complete prosthesis of
patellofemoral joint

that the pressure between femur and tibia when the knee is flexed to 45°
increased $4^1/_2 \times$ after a patellectomy.

Prosthesis: Prosthetic substitutions of the patellofemoral joint should be
considered for retropatellar arthrosis. McKeever [31] initially developed the
patellar prosthesis from Vitallium. Various patellar prostheses are available to
used in association with total knee replacements. Figure 16 illustrates the
Münster patella used with the Guepar knee. A newer product is the complete
prosthetic replacement of the patellofemoral joint which is supplied by Richards
(Fig. 17).

Just as the conservative procedures claim a success rate of 80%, most surgical procedures reported in the literature show a similar success rate. Insall [23] reported on 62 patients treated by drilling according to Pridie's method. Seventy-five percent were good or very good. Bentley [3] and West [3, 36] reported the same results in over 80% of their patellectomies. Dinham [8] reported 65% good results and Geckeler [15] 52%. Burton [5] who carefully assessed his patients observed only 35% good results following patellectomy and Scott [35] observed that only 5% had a good functional result. Hamacher [21] stressed that early patellectomy produces a better functional result than the same procedure done at a later stage.

Bandi [1] reported good and very good results in 60% of the forward displacement of the tibial tubercle. For the same procedure Nasseri [32] reported a 90% success rate.

Insall described 75% of patellar shavings as good, Chrisman [7] and Wiles [38] 70%, but Bentley described good results in only 45% of his cases, while Janssen [25] found no case of primary disturbances of the gliding surfaces.

It is often necessary to combine realignment and improvement of the gliding surface. For example, in a patient with recurrent dislocation of the patella and progressive degeneration of the articular surface, it will be necessary during the same procedure to realign the patella, smooth the articular surface, and reduce the retropatellar pressure. The key to success in the treatment of chondromalacia patellae lies in a combined procedure which can be best suited to the individual case, taking into account the etiology of the problem and improving the mechanical factors operating across the joint.

References

1. Bandi, W.: Chondromalazia patellae und femoro-patellare Arthrose. Helv. chir. Acta Suppl. **11,** (1972)
2. Baumgartl, F.: Das Kniegelenk. Berlin–Göttingen–Heidelberg–New York: Springer 1964
3. Bentley, G.: Chondromalacia patellae. J. Bone Jt. Surg. **52 A,** 221 (1970)
4. Blumensaat, C.: Die Lageabweichungen und Verrenkungen der Kniescheibe. Ergebn. Chir. **31,** 183 (1938)
5. Burton, V. W., Thomas, H. M.: Results of extension of the patella. Surg. Gynec. Obstet. **135,** 753 (1972)
6. Campbell, C.: Campbell's Operative Orthopaedics. St. Louis Mosby: 1971
7. Chrisman, O. D., Nook, G. A.: The role of patelloplasty and patellectomy in the arthritic knee, Chir. Orthop. **101,** 40 (1974)
8. Dinham, J. M., French, P. R.: Results of patellectomy for osteoarthritis. Postgrad. med. J. **48,** 590 (1972)
9. Eichler, J.: Die konservative Therapie der Gonarthrose. Z. Orthop. **111,** 516 (1973)
10. Ficat, P., Bizou, H.: Luxations récidivantes de la rotule. Rev. Orthop. **53,** 721 (1967)
11. Ficat, P., Philippe, J.: Zit. n. Ficat
12. Ficat, P., Philippe, J., Cuzaco, J. P., Cabrol, S., Belossi, J.: Le Syndrome d'hyperpression externe de la rotule (S.H.P.E!). Une entitie radioclinique. J. Radiol. Electrol. **53,** 845 (1972)
13. Ficat, P., Ficat, C., Bailleux, A.: Syndrome d'hyperpression externe de la rotule. Son intérét pour la connaissance de l'arthrose. Rev. Chir. orthop. **61,** 39 (1975)

14. Fürmaier, A.: Beitrag zur Mechanik der Patella und des Kniegelenkes. Arch. Orthop. Unfall-Chir. **46**, 78 (1953)
15. Geckeler, E. O., Quaranta, A. V.: Patellectomy for degenerative arthritis of the knee. J. Bone Jt. Surg. **44 A**, 1109 (1962)
16. Golthwait, J. E.: Permanent dislocation of the patella, Ann. Surg. **29**, 62 (1899)
17. Goymann, V., Bopp, H. M.: Chondrektomie und Gelenktoilette bei schweren Arthrosen des femurpatellaren Gleitweges. Z. Orthop. **111**, 534 (1973)
18. Green, W. T.: Quadricepsplasty in Treatment of Recurrent Subluxation of the Patella. Zit. nach Madigan
19. Groeneveld, H. B.: Neuere Möglichkeiten der Behandlung der femuro-patellaren Arthrose. Z. Orthop. **111**, 527 (1973)
20. Haglund, P.: Die hintere Patellakontusion. Zbl. Chir. **53**, 1757 (1926)
21. Hamacher, P.: Totale Patellektomie. Hefte Unfallheilk. **120**, 85 (1975)
22. Hauser, D. W.: Total tendon transplant for slipping patella. Surg. Gynec. Obstet. **66**, 199 (1938)
23. Insall, J.: The Pridie debridement operation for osteoarthritis of the knee. Clin. Orthop. **101**, 61 (1974)
24. Insall, J., Salvati, E.: Patella position in the normal knee joint. Radiology **101**, 101 (1971)
25. Hanssen, G.: Die Chondropathia patellae als Prägonarthrose. Zur Ätiologie und Therapie anhand von Ergebnissen nach Abrasio patellae. Z. Orthop. **112**, 1036 (1974)
26. Keyl, W., Viernstein, K.: Zur Behandlung bei Chondropathia patellae beim Sportler. Münch. med. Wschr. **31**, 1384 (1972)
27. Krogius, A.: Zur operativen Behandlung der habituellen Luxation der Patella. Zbl. Chir. **31**, 254 (1904)
28. Lee, K. J.: Kulturen embryonaler Knochenanlagen **in vitro** als Arbeitsmodell zum Studium von Pharmakaeinflüssen auf Bindegewebsfunktionen. Dissertation, Bonn 1972
29. Madigan, R., Wissinger, T., Donaldson, W.: Preliminary experience with a method of quadricepsplasty in recurrent subluxation of the patella, J. Bone Jt. Surg. **57 A**, 600. (1975)
30. Maquet, P.: Un traitement biomécanique de l'arthrose fémoropatelleire: L'avance-ment du tendon rotulien. Rev. Rhum. **30**, 779 (1963)
31. McKeever, D.: Patella prosthesis. J. Bone Jt. Surg. **37 A**, 1074 (1955)
32. Nasseri, D., Süssenbach, F.: Therapie der patellofemoralen Arthrose durch Ven-tralisierung der Tuberositas tibiae. Z. Orthop. **111**, 84 (1973)
33. Outerbridge, R. E.: The etiology of chondromalacia patellae. J. Bone Jt. Surg. **46 B**, 179 (1964)
34. Pridie, K. H.: A method of resurfacing osteoarthritic knee joint. J. Bone Jt. Surg. **41 B**, 618 (1959)
35. Scott, J. C.: Fractures of the patella. J. Bone Jt. Surg. **36 B**, 553 (1954)
36. West, E. E., Soto-Hall, R.: Recurrent dislocation of the patella in the adult. End results of patellectomy with quadricepsplasty. J. Bone Jt. Surg. **40 A**, 386 (1958)
37. Wiberg, G.: Roentgenographic and anatomic studies on the femoro-patellar joint with special reference to chondromalacia patellae. Acta Orthop. Scand. **12**, 319 (1941)
38. Wiles, Ph., Andrews, P. S., Bremer, R. A.: Chondromalacia of the patella. A study of later results of excision of the articular cartilage. J. Bone Jt. Surg. **42 B**, 65 (1960)

Translation from the German: Retropatellare Arthrose (Diagnose und Therapieüber-sicht). In: Knorpelschaden am Knie, 4. Reisensburger Workshop zur klinischen Unfall-chirurgie, edited by C. Burri and A. Rüter. In: Hefte zur Unfallheilkunde, Vol. 127 (1976). © Springer-Verlag 1976.

Patellar Shaving (Indications, Technique, Results)

H. R. Henche

Anatomy

In order to understand retropatellar damage, the anatomic peculiarities of the patellofemoral joint must be reviewed. The femur has two different large facets which articulate with the patella. The lateral is large and broad without a proximal marginal edge (Fig. 1). The medial is triangular, much smaller than the lateral, and provided with a sharp cartilaginous crest on the proximal end at the margin of the articular cartilage. Surfaces for the patella are separated from the condyle by a line which may be termed the "linea condylopatellaris". The lateral linea runs relatively horizontally while medially the cartilaginous crest rises

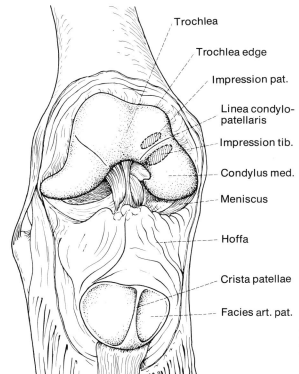

Trochlea

Trochlea edge

Impression pat.

Linea condylo-patellaris

Impression tib.

Condylus med.

Meniscus

Hoffa

Crista patellae

Facies art. pat.

Fig. 1. Knee joint with open patellofemoral joint. Particularly noteworthy are the two typical impressions above and below the medial linea condylopatellaris

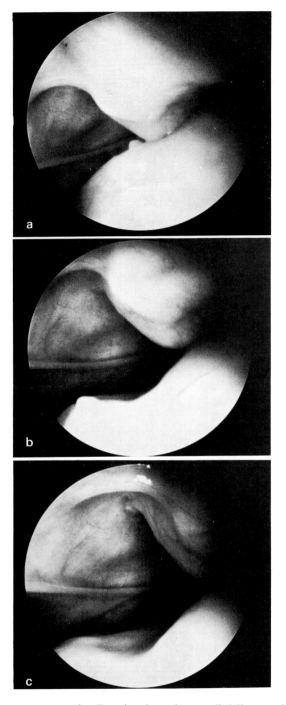

Fig. 2. (a) Arthroscopic picture of patellofemoral joint. The distal patellar edge is situated in the impression above the medial "linea condylopatellaris". (b) During flexion the patella leaves the impression. (c) At 90° of flexion the patella is situated in the upper portion of the trochlea. The impression located proximally to the "linea condylopatellaris" is not completely visible

more steeply. Proximal to the medial line an impression is borne by the lower patella margin (Fig. 2a–c). Distal to this line the medial condylar impression produced by the medial meniscus and anterior edge of tibia are located.

The patella is divided into two unequal halves by the crista patellae. The lateral side is large and flatly concave, while the medial facet is much smaller and not necessarily concave. Because of this the lateral contact within the patellofemoral joint has a large and relatively good surface while the medial contact is extremely variable and often small. Hüter [7], Mikulicz [13], von Meyer [12], May [11].

Anatomic variations in form of the patellofemoral joint can also be noted clinically and radiologically. Changes in the articular cartilage are frequently found when the patella is displaced upward. There is aplasia of the femoral condyle, genu valgum or various abnormal patellar shapes as described by Wiberg [18] and Baumgartl [1]. Braune and Fischer [3] have proposed the theory that the articular cartilage is especially thick where large articular incongruities are present. If the physiologic incongruity is aggravated by anatomic alterations, then cartilage damage can be expected as a result of either a disturbance of the nutritional supply or an increased predisposition to microtrauma.

Traumatic Cartilage Lesions

In addition to anatomic abnormalities trauma may cause chondromalacia patellae. Direct cartilage damage is most obvious in patellar fracture. Even after the bone has healed the articular cartilage damage remains. If the fracture is caused by flexion, then the articular damage is relatively minor. On the other hand, contusion produces extensive damage and often enzymatic disintegration of the cartilage continues independently and results in extensive chondromalacia patellae. The diagnosis is more difficult in the case of a pure cartilage fracture.

The most common injuries to the patellofemoral joint are contusions without fracture. This results in destruction of the cartilage cells and a release of proteolytic enzymes from the lysosomes. According to Chrisman [4] the cathepsin D complex plays the decisive role in the enzymatic cartilage destruction which follows. The proof that enzymes can damage cartilage was provided by Puhl [16] based on scanning electron microscopy investigations. This autolytic process causes a synovitis of the knee joint. This in turn can be held responsible for the patient's pain.

Osteoarthrosis and Hemarthrosis

Due to enzyme activity, chronic effusions caused by various infections or hemathroses may damage the articular cartilage so that erosions appear on the articular surface. The damage to the articular cartilage may be so severe that a return to normal is not possible [14, 9].

Clinical Symptoms of Chondromalacia Patellae

When the condition is not traumatic it usually begins at a young age. Girls are affected three times more frequently than boys. The symptoms are as follows: The patient complains of a dull ache in the entire knee joint. With prolonged weight-bearing the knee frequently gives way without cause. Stiffness with sitting is common and the patients sense the need to frequently move their knees. Climbing stairs increases the pain. Chondromalacia patellae produces pain on descending a hill or stairs and frequently feelings of weakness or cramping in the quadriceps are experienced. It is common for chondromalacia to appear 3 to 4 months after an injury such as a direct contusion.

Clinical Examination

Synovial thickening is fairly frequent. Small synovial pads protrude on each side of the patellar tendon. These are easily seen when the quadriceps are tightened. In the seated position a patella alta is especially obvious, resulting in the so-called "pointed knee."

Palpation of the patella often reveals tenderness to pressure over the medial patellar facet. Both facets can be palpated by moving the patella from side to side (Fig. 3). This can also determine whether dislocation or subluxation is the cause of the chondromalacia. When the quadriceps is tightened, the movement of the patella should be observed. Normally it moves proximally, but a lateral movement indicates a tendency for subluxation. Suprapatellar pressure with quadriceps contraction may produce typical pain as described by Zohlan. This finding should not be overemphasized as it may be painful even in a healthy

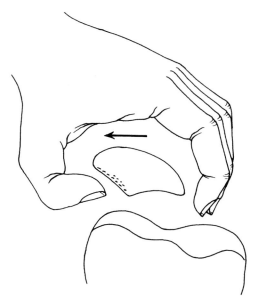

Fig. 3. By medial displacement of the patella the medial patellar facet can be examined by the thumb and tested for sensitivity to pressure

joint. Mobility is usually normal, but there is often palpable or audible crepitus deep to the patella. Intensity of the crepitus increases when the weight-bearing joint is flexed. Frequently a snapping of the patella is observed at 30°−40° of flexion. This occurs most commonly when the linea condylopatellaris is more prominent.

X-ray Examination

In painful knees we normally carry out a standard radiological examination consisting of one AP, one lateral, one oblique, and three tangential or skyline views, with the knee flexed at 30°, 60° and 90°. When the diagnosis is chondromalacia we pay special attention to the height of the patella. In 30° of flexion the inferior pole of the patella should not be located more than one cm above Blumensaat line [8]. In the lateral X-ray special attention is paid to the Haglund excavation. This sclerotic area in the middle of the patella is not a sure indication of chondromalacia since it is frequently seen in normal knees. In our opinion, the Haglund excavation is caused by the cartilage-bone crest in the region of the proximal, medial, femoral condyle as described by Outerbridge [15]. The shape of the patella in the tangential view is more important. In reviewing recurrent dislocations [6], we observed the patella type IV of Wiberg and Baumgartl in 65% of our cases. In 6% of the cases, the so-called "Hunter's cap" shape was seen. Normally these two variants are only found in 40% of patellae according to Bengert [2].

Conservative Treatment

The usual methods of physical therapy can be used in the treatment of the reactive synovitis. Because of the encouraging reports of Chrisman [5] and Volastro [17] we have attempted to administer salicylates over a period of several weeks. The salicylates are said to restrain the enzyme complexes responsible for cartilage destruction. We did not achieve any clear clinical results. Injections of steroids and other medications have also been unsuccessful.

Surgical Treatment

Most cases are treated by patellar shave in conjunction with other procedures, such as transplantation of the tibial tubercle. The indication for patellar shave alone is based on previous arthroscopy (Fig. 4). The diagnosis of the stage of chondromalacia patellae is not possible on clinical and X-ray examinations. The necessity for surgery can be determined by arthroscopic examination.

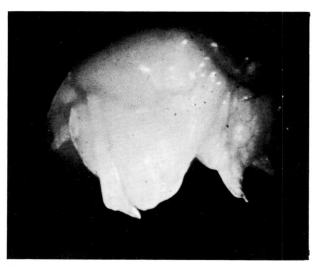

Fig. 4. Arthroscopic picture of a severe chondropathia patellae with almost complete degeneration of the articular cartilage

The operative technique is simple. A medial parapatellar incision is used. It must be large enough so that the patella can be exposed in all areas. An ulcerlike defect is frequently found on the medial facet. The edges of the cartilage are usually undermined.

First, using a normal scalpel the margins of the ulcer are defined and the overhanging cartilage removed. Once the surgeon is convinced a firm connection exists between the cartilage and the subchondral bone at the ulcer edge, the entire floor can be cleaned using a sharp curette or scalpel. All gelantinoid cartilage must be removed. Usually the floor of the ulcer extends to the subchondral bone. If this is the case, multiple drill holes are made so that granulation tissue can grow from the cancellous bone. This is essential for healing of the facet. Should the cartilage ulcer not extend to the subchondral bone, we perforate the base from outside of the articular surface.

When closing, a medial capsulorrhaphy is almost always performed. This is done to increase the contact surface of the medial patellofemoral joint.

Results of Patellar Shaving

Between 1965 and 1974 we performed arthrotomies on 60 patients, in whom only a patellar shave was done. We are not including combined procedures in this evaluation. The average age was 26 years and women outnumbered men by 3.5 to 1. Trauma was implicated in 72%, usually a direct contusion. A medium to severe reactive synovitis was present in all cases.

A questionnaire was sent to all patients and 58 responded. 30% are completely symptom free, 78% report a significant improvement, and 60%

feel that they have more security in their knee. 88% consider the operation successful, but 70% still have some complaints. Inability to sit without pain for prolonged periods is the most common. Fourteen of the sixty patients are still undergoing treatment for their problem.

Conclusion

The source of damage to the deep surface of the patella can be based on many causes. The incongruity of this joint combined with the unusual thickness of the articular cartilage is a major factor. While investigating the nutritional supply, Marondas [10] determined the cartilage up to a thickness of 3 mm can be adequately nourished with glucose if the pressure is alternated. In the absence of pressure or in the case of constant pressure, nutrition is poor and the cartilage is only nourished for a distance of about 1.7 mm. Anatomic variations such as the patellar forms described by Wiberg and Baumgartl can promote chondromalacia patellae as well. Fractures, massive contusions, and chronic effusions lead to destruction of the superficial cartilage layer and the release of enzyme complexes.

To date no sure medication has been found to deter enzymatic destruction of articular cartilage or encourage regeneration.

Patellar shaving has been judged successful by almost 90% of our patients. This is encouraging since the procedure represents a form of therapeutic help-lessness.

We are not in a position to determine the difference between conservative and surgical treatment in adults. In investigating the course of chondromalacia patella in childhood Steinbrecher stated that after one year 63% of the surgically treated patients were symptom free while only 23% of the nonoperative patients were comfortable. We feel patellar shaving reduces the period of pain and promotes quicker recovery. Our present knowledge suggests that medication will not cure this condition.

Summary

The anatomy of the patellofemoral joint is briefly described. The causes of chon-dromalacia patellae are classified into anatomic variations in form and various types of trauma. Chronic synovitis and recurrent effusions are capable of dam-aging the articular surface through enzymatic processes. The clinical picture of chondromalacia patella is presented. During the physical examination it is especially important to note the location of the patella and its pattern of move-ment. Pain on compression of the patella and local tenderness over the patellar facet are significant findings.

Various patellar forms should be observed on radiological examination. Conservative treatment is usually lengthy and promises little success. In over 60 isolated cases of patellar shaving, 88% judged the operation successful after one year. Fourteen patients still have residual complaints. The overall results of patellar shaving must be considered good.

References

1. Baumgartl, F. A.: Das Kniegelenk. Berlin–Göttingen–Heidelberg–New York: Springer 1964
2. Bengert, O.: Beitrag zur Chondropathia patellae. Arch. orthop. Unfall-Chir. **56,** 458 (1964)
3. Braune, W., Fischer, O.: Die Bewegungen des Kniegelenkes. Nach einer neuen Methode am lebenden Menschen. Abhandl. kgl. Sächs. Ges. Wiss. II, Bd. **XVII,** S. 77 ff., Leipzig 1891
4. Chrisman, O. D.: Biochemical aspects of degenerative joint disease. Clin. Orthop. **64,** 77 (1969)
5. Chrisman, O. D., Snook, G. A., Wilson, T. C.: The protective effect of aspirin against degeneration of human articular cartilage. Clin. Orthop. **84,** 193 (1972)
6. Henche, H. R.: Klinik und Therapie der Chondropathia patellae. Ther. Umschau **30,** 255 (1973)
7. Hüter, C.: Anatomische Studien an den Extremitätengelenken Neugeborener und Erwachsener. Das Kniegelenk. Virchows Arch. path. Anat. **26,** 484 (1863)
8. Jacobsen, K., Bertheussen, K.: The vertical location of the patella. Acta Orthop. Scand. **45,** 436 (1974)
9. Mankin, H. J.: Localisation of tritiated thymidine in articular cartilage of rabbits. J. Bone Jt. Surg. **45 A,** 529 (1963)
10. Marondas, A. et al.: The permeability of articular cartilage. J. Bone Jt. Surg. **50 B,** 166 (1968)
11. May, E. et al.: Knorpelläsionen an den Femurcondylen im Experiment bei Traumatisierung der Patella. Arch. orthop. Unfall-Chir. **54,** 301 (1962)
12. Meyer von, H.: Der Mechanismus der Kniescheibe. Arch. Anat. **280** (1880)
13. Mikulicz, J.: Über individuelle Formdifferenzen am Femur und an der Tibia des Menschen. Arch. Anat., **351** (1878)
14. Otta, P.: Über das Wachstum des Gelenkknorpels. Heidelberg: Hüthig 1965
15. Outerbridge, R. E.: Further studies on the etiology of chondromalacia patellae. J. Bone Jt. Surg. **46 B,** 179 (1964)
16. Puhl, W., Dustmann, H. O., Schulitz, K. P.: Knorpelveränderungen bei experimentellen Hämarthros. Z. Orthop. **109,** 475 (1971)
17. Volastro, P. S., Malawista, S. E., Chrisman, O. D.: Protective and destructive effects on injured rabbit cartilage in vivo. Clin. Orthop. **91,** 243 (1973)
18. Wiberg, G.: Mechanisch funktionelle Faktoren der Arthrosis deformans in Hüft- und Kniegelenk. Z. Orthop. **75,** 260 (1944)

Translation from the German: Abrasio patellae (Indikation, Technik, Ergebnisse). In: Knorpelschaden am Knie, 4. Reisensburger Workshop zur klinischen Unfallchirurgie, edited by C. Burri and A. Rüter. In: Hefte zur Unfallheilkunde, Vol. 127 (1976). © Springer-Verlag 1976.

Retinacular Release
(Indications, Technique, Results)

D. Baumann and L. Leichs

Chondromalacia patellae [2] represents a lesion of the posterior surface of the patella for which three stages can be distinguished; cartilage edema, the appearance of fissures, and finally the erosion of cartilage down to subchondral bone accompanied by peeling of scaly cartilaginous pieces. Autopsy investigations [17] showed that with increasing age the appearance of chondromalacic foci increased. In 33% of the arthrotomies undertaken for meniscus lesions, chondromalacic foci were also found. A high percentage of chondropathic alterations, therefore, exist without clinical symptoms.

An external cause is necessary to transform the latent form into symptomatic chondromalacia patellae. Clinical symptoms are promoted by direct (contusions and fractures) and indirect (twisting) trauma [1, 3, 8, 11, 20]. Dysplasias and lateral subluxations of the patella as well as dysplasias of the femoral condyles favor chondromalacia patellae. This leads to a disturbed pattern of movement of the patellofemoral facet with a tilting of the patella [6]. This in turn leads to a syndrome of lateral hypercompression caused by the predominance of the lateral structures (vastus lateralis and iliotibial tract) over the often atrophic vastus medialis (Fig. 1). Through the lateral release of the retinaculum, the preponderance of the lateral forces and the tilting of the patella should be eliminated. Through simultaneous medial release of the retinaculum — carefully protecting the insertion of the vastus medialis — the medial attachment of the patella is also lifted.

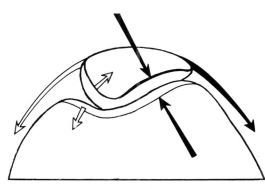

Fig. 1. Lateral hypercompression syndrome (according to Ficat)

Materials and Methods

Between January 1970 and 1975, we performed releases of the retinaculum in 53 patients, 48 of those patients were available for follow-up examination. We were able to include 57 knees in the statistics as nine patients had bilateral procedures. Table 1 shows the radiographic findings for the 57 knees. The distribution of the patellar types corresponds to the norm. A bipartite patella was found in two patients, a patella alta according to the index devised by Insall and Salvati [10] in three patients, and Haglund's impression in 21 knees. The hypercompression syndrome accompanied by tilting of the patella and subchondral sclerosis was found in 32 knees, a subluxation in eight, a patellofemoral arthrosis in 13, a fracture of the patella in 2, Sudeck's disease in one, and 15 patients exhibited osteoporosis. A femoral dysplasia measured according to Brattström's angular aperture [5] was observed in five patients. We found ten cases of an Outerbridge ridge and slight osteoarthrosis in five knee joints.

The shape of the patella and the distal femur determines the direction of the pressure forces appearing in the patellofemoral facet. The more the medial patellar joint facet is reduced in size and the flatter the medial condyle becomes, the larger the laterally directed pressure forces become (Fig. 2). The quotient for the length of the patellar tendon and the diameter of the patella is usually 1 [10]. A quotient of 1.3 has been set as the upper limit for the standard (Fig. 3).

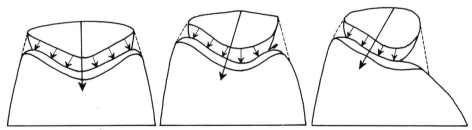

Fig. 2. Variations in form of the patellofemoral joint with resulting pressures

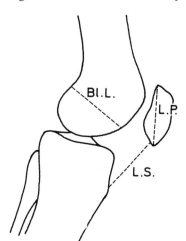

Fig. 3. Determination of the patellar height L. S. (length of the patellar tendon) to L. P. (longitudinal diameter of the patella) is 1 (Insall and Salvati)

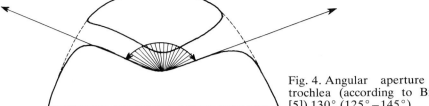

Fig. 4. Angular aperture of the trochlea (according to Brattström [5]) 130° (125° – 145°)

The lateral hypercompression syndrome [6] consists in a lateral tilting of the patella accompanied by widening of the medial and narrowing of the lateral interarticular space. At an angular aperture of more than 145°, dysplasia of the distal femoral condyles exists [5] (Fig. 4).

We made the clinical diagnosis of chondromalacia patellae based on the patellar symptoms of spontaneous retropatellar pain and the provoked pain such as tenderness of the facets, pain on suprapatellar pressure, pain on percussion of the patella, and the hypercompression symptoms caused by prolonged sitting or climbing stairs were all taken into consideration. Table 2 lists the pre- and post-operative complaints. Table 3 lists the secondary complaints.

Table 1. X-ray findings on 57 knees with chondropathia patellae

Patella type	
Wiberg I	8 (14.3%)
Wiberg II	33 (7.0%)
Wiberg II/III	8 (14.3%)
(Baumgartl)	
Wiberg III	6 (10.7%)
Wiberg IV	2 (3.7%)
Bipartite patella	2
Patella alta (index according to Insall/Salvati larger than 1.3)	3
Haglund's impression	21
Hypercompression syndrome (tilting of the patella, subchondral sclerosis)	32
Subluxation	8
Patellofemoral arthrosis	13
Fracture	2
Sudeck's atrophy	1
Osteoporosis	15
Dysplasia of the femur (angular aperture according to Brattström more than 145°)	5
Outerbridge ridge	10
Arthrosis of the knee	5

Table 2. Pre- and postoperative clinical picture of chondromalacia patellae in 57 knees

	Preop	Postop	Improve-ment
Spontaneous retropatellar pain	57	12	23
Provoked pains			
Tenderness of the facets	49	3	23
Pain on suprapatellar pressure	51	3	21
Percussion of patella Hypercompression	51	3	23
Prolonged sitting	48	9	13
Climbing stairs	52	7	15

Table 3. Pre- and postoperative clinical picture of chondromalacia patellae in 57 knees (secondary complaints)

	Preop	Postop
Crepitus	54	52
Compression	8	0
Effusion	11	1
Atrophy larger than 2 cm	23	14
Giving way	9	2
Sign of meniscus	11	0
Ligament laxity	4	1

Results

Upon questioning, 33 patients (58%) stated that they were very satisfied with the result of the operation, i.e., they were again able to participate in physical activities and pursue their occupations, and after prolonged periods of weight-bearing suffered no complaints. Ten patients (17.5%) were just satisfied with the result, i.e., they ⸱uffered occasional complaints after more intense weight-bearing as a result of physical or occupational activities. On the other hand, 14 patients (24.5%) were dissatisfied with the result of the operation, i.e., no improvement of the preoperative complaints was achieved. These patients were occupationally handicapped.

To objectively evaluate the results the patients were divided into three groups. Group I consisted of those patients who subjectively and objectively were without complaints; group II consisted of those patients with slight to moderate complaints of patellar origin, and group III consisted of those with complaints unimproved by the operation. Group I had 29 patients (50%) group II had 13 patients (23%) and group III had 15 patients (27%).

The patients in Group III were put through special clinical and radiological assessments. The radiological evaluation revealed a higher percentage of patellar types III and IV according to Wiberg's classification system and a higher percentage of femoral dysplasias. Half of the patients with patellofemoral arthrosis also exhibited poor results and both patients with old patellar fractures remained in pain.

We, therefore, consider a release of the retinacula to be indicated when conservative therapy fails, in the case of a clinically definitive diagnosis based on the typical patellar symptoms, crepitus and atrophy, radiological signs of the lateral hypercompression syndrome, and with no radiographic signs of dysplasia or patellofemoral arthrosis. A release of the retinacula is contraindicated in the case of dysplasia of the patella (types III and IV Wiberg's classification) and dysplasias of the distal femoral condyle. Secondary changes in the patel femoral joint such as arthrosis or old fracture are also contraindications to release of the retinacula. Associated ligament instabilities should take precedence over chondromalacia. Sudeck's atrophy is also a contraindication to operation.

Release of the retinacula offers the following advantages: It is a minor operation which can be carried out simultaneously on both sides. Postoperative convalescence is minimal. Further surgical measures can still be undertaken. The 73% good or satisfactory results support the method. Healing of the cartilage lesion can probably only be expected in stage I, the edema stage, while in the case of advanced cartilage lesions, only a transformation of a manifest disease into a clinically latent stage can be achieved.

References

1. Aleman, O.: Chondromalacia posttraumatica patellae, Acta chir. scand. **63,** 149 (1928)
2. Büdinger, K.: Über Ablösung von Gelenkteilen und verwandt. Prozesse. Dtsch. Z. Chir. **84,** 311 (1906)
3. Bandi, W.: Chondromalacia patellae und femoro-patellare Arthrose. Helvetia Chirurgica Acta, Suppl. **11,** Basel: Schwabe 1972
4. Baumgartl, F.: Das Kniegelenk. Berlin–Göttingen–Heidelberg–New York: Springer 1964
5. Brattström, H.: Shape of the intercondylar groove normally and in recurrent dislocation of the patella. Acta chir. scand. Suppl. **68,** 1
6. Ficat, P.: Pathologie femoro-patellaire. Paris: Masson Cie., 1970
7. Fürmeier, A.: Beitrag zur Ätiologie der Chondropathia patellae Arch. orthop. Unfall-Chir. **46,** 178 (1953)
8. Haglund, P.: Die hintere Patellacontusion. Zbl. Chir. **53,** 1757 (1926)
9. Henche, H. R.: Klinik und Therapie der Chondropathia patellae. Therap. Umschau, Band **30,** Heft 3 (1973)
10. Insall, J., Salvati, E.: Patella position in the normal knee joint. Radiology **101,** 101 (1971)
11. Karlsson, S.: Chondromalacia patellae. Acta chir. scand. **83,** 347 (1939)
12. Keyl, W., Viernstein, K.: Zur Behandlung der Chondropathia patellae beim Sportler. Münch. med. Wsch. **31,** 1384 (1972)
13. Lnutson, F.: Über die Röntgenologie des Femoropatellargelenkes sowie eine gute Projektion des Kniegelenkes. Acta radiol. (Stockholm) **22,** 371 (1941)
14. Maquet, P.: Biomechanische Aspekte der Femur-Patella Beziehungen. Z. Orthop. **112,** 620 (1974)

15. Merchant, A., et al.: Roentgenographic analysis of patellofemoral congruence. J. Bone Jt. Surg. **56 A,** 1391 (1974)
16. Outerbridge, R. E.: The etiology of chondromalacia patellae. J. Bone Jt. Surg. **43 B,** 752 (1961)
17. Owre, A.: Chondromalacia Patellae. Acta chir. scand. Vol. **77,** Suppl. 41 (1936)
18. Rohlederer, O.: Ätiologie und Symptomatologie der Präluxatio Patellae. Zbl. Chir. **76,** I. 103 (1951)
19. Silfverskiöld, N.: Chondromalacia of the patella. Acta orthop. scand. **9,** 214 (1938)
20. Viernstein, K., Weigert, M.: Chondromalazia patellae beim Leistungssportler. Z. Orthop. **104,** 432 (1968)
21. Wiberg, G.: Roentgenographic and anatomic studies on the femoropatellar joint. Acta Orthop. Scand. **12,** 319 (1941)
22. Wiles, P., et al.: Chondromalacia patellae. J. Bone Jt. Surg. **38 B,** 95 (1956)

Translation from the German: Retinaculumspaltung (Indikation, Technik, Ergebnisse). In: Knorpelschaden am Knie, 4. Reisensburger Workshop zur klinischen Unfallchirurgie, edited by C. Burri and A. Rüter: In: Hefte zur Unfallheilkunde, Vol. 127 (1976). © Springer-Verlag 1976.

Anterior Displacement of the Tibial Tuberosity

W. Bandi

Introduction

Every lesion of articular hyaline cartilage can lead to arthrosis. It deserves, therefore, our diagnostic attention and therapeutic endeavors. One of the most frequent cartilage lesions of the knee is chondromalacia patellae (CP). It is, in our opinion, more frequent than meniscal lesions and is significant in the pathogenesis of osteoarthrosis of the knee.

Characteristics of Chondromalacia Patellae

Chondromalacia patellae exhibits three stages of severity:
Stage 1: localized yellowish-brown discoloration and dullness of the cartilage accompanied by loss of elasticity
Stage 2: splitting and fissuring of the cartilage, with cartilaginous desquamation into the synovial cavity with reactive synovitis
Stage 3: ulcerous degeneration of the cartilage with exposed, sclerotic, subchondral bone and ingrowth of a pannus on the patellar joint surface. Vascular connective tissue grows from the medullary space into the degenerate, basal cartilage layer and leads to the formation of osteophytes and the transition to arthrosis.
Physically, a reduction in elasticity can be measured in these regions.
Chemically, a reduction in the content of chondroitin-sulfuric acid can be measured not only in the superficial but also in the deeper zones.
Histologically, the collagenous fibrils become visible in the intercellular substance (unmasked), and at stage 1 the chondrocytes exhibit signs of proliferation, whereas at stages 2 and 3 increasing signs of disintegration appear.
Functionally, the loss in elasticity results in an impairment of the nutritional supply since the massaging action necessary for diffusion no longer is adequate. Simultaneously, the friction coefficient increases with the increase in mechanical wear. Destructive and nutritional disturbances intensify themselves in a vicious circle.

Clinical Picture of Chondromalacia Patellae

Chondromalacia patellae occurs more frequently than previously assumed (Aleman [1], Owre [14], Crooks [7], Fründ [10], De Montomollin [12], Outerbridge [13], Schneider [15], Viernstein [16]. The lesion of the patellar cartilage found frequently at autopsy permits the assumption that many of these cases heal spontaneously by forming a solid fibrocartilage without becoming clinically manifest. If trauma occurs during this latent stage, it leads to the *immediate* symptom picture of retropatellar damage, quite in contrast to those cases where trauma affects a *healthy* patellar articular cartilage. Here one observes that the initial traumatic pain subsides and only after a latent period of 6−12 weeks does the symptom picture of chondromalacia appear. Since mechanical damage to healthy articular cartilage leads to a complete picture of chondromalacia patellae only after several weeks, the correct interpretation of this latent period is important for the written professional opinion concerning the accident.

While patellofemoral arthrosis can be decisively diagnosed radiologically, the diagnosis of chondromalacia patellae is more difficult. The symptomatic picture is summarized by Ficat [8] under the name *patellar syndrome.*

1. *Spontaneous pain:* localized under the patella, occasionally on its medial edge, and sometimes over the medial joint line (contusion with meniscal damage)

2. *Provoked pain:* Pain during palpation of the patellar joint surface when the patella is shifted medially or laterally (probably caused by the inflamed synovium)

Pain experienced by a blow to the patella when the knee joint is flexed (Fründ's sign, not reliable).

Zohlen's sign [17]: pain experienced when the patella (which is pressed posteriorly by the investigator) is pulled upward when the patient's straight leg rises.

Hypercompression pain: A retropatellar pain, which is static during sitting and dynamic during ascending and descending stairs.

Standing-up phenomenon: When standing up from a deep knee bend with the upper part of the body simultaneously bent forward, there is relatively little pain, whereas when the same movement is carried out with the upper part of the body erect, i.e., the body weight displaced backward, there is significantly more pain [2].

3. *Reduction of gliding ability:* Crepitus and giving-way, sudden collapse of the knee joint when climbing stairs, or occasionally when walking on a level surface may occur.

The hypercompression signs, especially Zohlen's sign, the standing-up phenomenon, and the retropatellar friction and giving-way have proven reliable.

Diagnostic Significance of X-Rays

The position of the patella with regard to its height on the lateral view and its centering between the femoral condyles on the A–P should be evaluated. The tangential X-rays of the patellofemoral joint when it is flexed at angles of 30°, 60°, and 90° are important.

Dysplasia of the patella according to Wiberg's types III and IV (Hunter's cap patella) and the flat, so-called gravel stone patella indirectly imply chondromalacia. Lateralization of the patella is usually accompanied by an overloading of the lateral facet and, as a result of insufficient counterpressure and poor massaging, by degenerative cartilage changes on the medial facet. Therefore, one can frequently recognize a clear lateral narrowing of the interarticular space and secondary manifestations of degeneration (calcification, formation of osteophytes on the medial facet or on the edge of the medial condyle). A further indirect sign of chondromalacia patellae is the stringy structure of the patellar trabecullae which resembles the radiological picture presented by Sudeck's atrophy.

Every radiological examination of the knee joint should include at least one tangential X-ray, especially when evaluating traumatic injuries. Occasionally one finds a crest fracture of the patella with secondary degenerative changes which would otherwise have been invisible.

Pathogenesis

The pathogenesis of chondromalacia patellae is difficult to recognize. It has the picture of degenerative cartilage change, but it is not uncommonly the result of a single injury. The following process is compatible with cartilage construction and clinical observations.

The primary lesion occurs in the tangential fibers of the hyaline articular cartilage and disturbs its structure, which according to Benninghoff is a prerequisite for its function. This results in a loss of elasticity, increase in the friction coefficient, and a reduction in the nutritional supply. The superficial tangential layer can be damaged by shear injury, by continuous pressure or enzymatically (hemarthrosis, inflammatory exudate). A disturbance in the nutritional supply can be caused by a lack of pressure and a lack of the massaging action of the cartilage (resting damage). Table 1 presents a survey of the possible pathogenic influences. Many of the factors presented in Table 1 have as a common denominator an overly high patellofemoral pressure. Although Ficat attempts to exclude those factors which are caused by defective positions in the frontal plane, we feel that the increased femoral pressure is the general cause of the damage [2]. Before going into details of therapy, I would like to illustrate the pathogenic significance of patella alta.

Table 1. Pathogenesis of chondromalacia patellae and patellofemoral arthrosis

Mechanical overstrain			Disturbed regeneration
Exogenous (trauma)		Endogenous	
Direct	Indirect		
Acute: Cartilage: Contusion Rupture (shearing-off) Bone: Fracture Patella Condyles } stage	Acute: Twist Hemarthrosis Posttraumatic fixation and stiffness	Dysplasia of the patella Wiberg III Patella parva, magna, partita	1. Alteration of synovia infection, hematogenous, *posttraumatic* autotoxic autoimmune reaction: PCP
Shaft Condyles Tibia head } defective position of axis and rotation		Defective position of patella Lateralization Chronic subluxation Recurrent dislocation	2. Alteration of circulation arteriosclerosis thrombosis neurogenous Sudeck's d. 3. Endocrine post-climacteric Osteoporosis Hypothyroid
Chronic: Overstrain Sports Occupational Weight	Chronic: posttraumatic neuromuscular causes posttraumatic Sudeck's d.	Patella alta Dysplasia of femoral condyles medial stage Rotation defect	

Joint Mechanics of Patella Alta

We classify as patella alta a patella whose apex is above Blumensaat's [6] line when the knee joint is flexed at an angle of 50°. This line is the continuation of a radiologic al density in the body of the condyles which corresponds to the cortex at the base of the intercondylar fossa. (Blumensaat himself set this line when the knee joint is flexed at an angle of 30°.) According to our observations, however, patella alta would then be extraordinarily frequent. In order to avoid borderline cases, therefore, we have chosen stricter terms for its definition (Fig. 1). In our opinion, patella alta causes a patellofemoral pressure increase. This is supported by the following:

1. Haglund's impression which often accompanies patella alta, an excavation and sclerosis in the patellar joint surface
2. The frequent occurrence of patella alta among our patients. In our cases of *100 patients* with chondromalacia patellae and patellofemoral arthrosis, we found 40% with patella alta. In a group with the same average age *without knee complaints,* we found only 20% with patella alta (10 for every 50 cases)

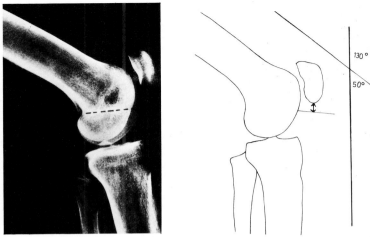

Fig. 1. Modification of Blumensaat's criteria for determining a patella alta (see text)

Joint Mechanics

By definition, when the knee joint is flexed at a comparable angle, patella alta is located higher in front of the condyles than the normal patella. Therefore, the angle between the quadriceps tendon and the ligamentum patellae becomes smaller, the results in the parallelogram of the pressure forces longer, and the patellofemoral pressure larger. In addition, when the knee joint is hyperflexed, the quadriceps tendon is entwined around the femoral condyles. In this manner, a portion of extension force proceeds as pressure on the femoral condyles and relieves the patellofemoral joint. We call this phenomenon the entwining effect. In the case of patella alta, this entwining effect appears later than in the case of a normal patella. Especially when the knee joint is hyperflexed, therefore, the patellofemoral joint is loaded with larger pressure forces (see also 11). Both in the experiment with a model and by calculating the entwining effect, an additional pressure of 20–40% was measured for patella alta.

Model Experiment: Models were made according to X-rays of a knee before and after correcting the position of the alta. The geometric relationships are determined by vertical photography at varying degrees of flexion and the patellofemoral pressure values calculated according to the following formula:

$$D = \frac{2Mq}{r} \cdot (\cos \frac{\gamma}{2} \cos \frac{\beta}{2})$$

q = body weight
r = lever arm of the extension apparatus at the knee joint
γ = angle formed by the quadriceps tendon and the ligamentum patellae
β = angle in the quadriceps tendon at entwining
M = muscle force · lever arm at the femur and lower leg (2)

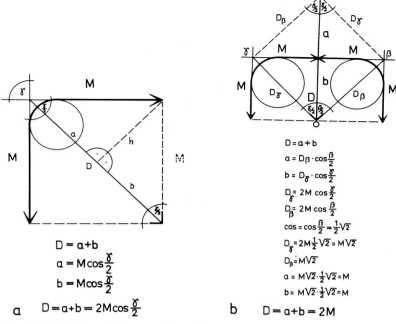

Fig. 2. Calculation of the entwining effect

Calculation of the Entwining Effect: If 2 weights M are hung on a string which is fed over a pulley, the pressure on this pulley is 2M cos $\frac{\gamma}{2}$ whereby γ is the angle enclosed by the string ends (Fig. 2a). If the string is fed over 2 pulleys, then the pressure on pulley 1 is 2M cos $\frac{\gamma}{2}$ and on pulley 2 is 2M cos $\frac{\beta}{2}$, whereby γ and β are the angles enclosed by the string ends. If the pulleys are situated symmetrically, then their pressure is the sum of both pressures (Fig. 2b), but if they are asymmetric, then the pressures are added according to the parallelogram of forces (Fig. 3a). According to this calculation, when the knee joint is flexed at an angle of 78° (as measured on X-ray), a ratio of 1:1.34 is obtained for the patellofemoral pressure values when the patella is at a normal position and at an alta position. Patella alta, therefore, produces an increase in pressure of 34%, a value of the same order as in the model experiment.

Treatment

The common pathogenic denominator for chondromalacia and patellofemoral arthrosis, whatever the cause may be, is generally or locally increased patellofemoral pressure. The reduction of this pressure represents effective therapy.

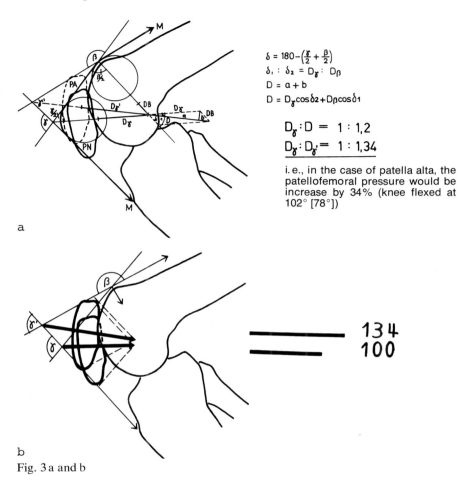

$$\delta = 180 - \left(\frac{\gamma}{2} + \frac{\beta}{2}\right)$$

$$\delta_1 : \delta_2 = D_\gamma : D_\beta$$

$$D = a + b$$

$$D = D_\gamma \cos\delta_2 + D_\beta \cos\delta_1$$

$$D_\gamma : D = 1 : 1,2$$

$$D_\gamma : D_\gamma' = 1 : 1,34$$

i.e., in the case of patella alta, the patellofemoral pressure would be increase by 34% (knee flexed at 102° [78°])

$$\frac{134}{100}$$

a

b

Fig. 3a and b

We attempt to reduce this pressure by improving the torque, i.e., lengthening the lever arm of the extension musculature. We have substantiated this therapy based on the mechanics of the joint. Figure 4 illustrates the results of calculations based on a model (not taking the entwining effect into consideration) and injuries to an autopsied knee carried out together with I. Brennwald. The forward displacement of the tibial tuberosity by 10 mm results in a reduction in pressure of 20%−40% in the patellofemoral joint [2].

Surgical Technique (Fig. 5): With a lateral parapatellar incision, the joint is widely exposed and inspected. Malacic cartilage and osteophytes are removed. Depending on the findings, other measures are undertaken (menisectomy, synovectomy, etc.). The synovial membrane is then closed and the fibrous capsule sutured only up to the level of the superior pole, distally it remains open to the ligamentum patellae. After the tibial tuberosity has been exposed, it is

Table 2. Cases

No. = 100	Average age	Period of postop. observation	Hospital stay (days)
♂ 56	52 years	∅ 5 years	∅ 27
♀ 44	(19–75)	(8.5–3)	(12–82)

Table 3. Operations on knee

Anterior displacement of tibial tuberosity	100
Shaving of cartilage (CP II and III GR)	89
Meniscectomy	21
Synovectomy	18
Osteotomy	16

Table 4. Complications

Resorption of (carina) – chip	2
Hematoma	3
Secondary healing over tibial tub.	1
Transitory pain at tibial tub.	3
Insufficient anterior displacement	1
	10

Table 5. Results

	No. = 100
Good (1–1.4)	70
Moderate (1.5–1.9)	18
Unchanged (2)	6
Poor (> 2)	6

Table 6. Changes in the subjective and objective results during the observation period of 5 years

			No. = 100
1	Increase in arthrosis Increase in complaints	↑↑	12
2	Increase in arthrosis Complaints remain constant	↑→	18
3	Increase in arthrosis Decrease in complaints	↑↓	10
4	Arthrosis remains constant Increase in complaints	→↑	2
5	Arthrosis remains constant Complaints remain constant	→	30
6	Arthrosis remains constant Decrease in complaints	→↓	24
7	Decrease in arthrosis Complaints remain constant	↓→	2
8	Decrease in arthrosis Decrease in complaints	↓↓	2

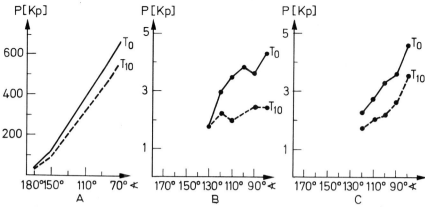

Fig. 4. Patellofemoral pressure values before and after displacement of the tibial tuberosity
A: Calculated according to formula
B: Measured on the model
C: Measured on autopsied knee
(T_0: tub. tibiae in situ. T_{10}: tub. tibiae tipped ventrally by 10 mm)

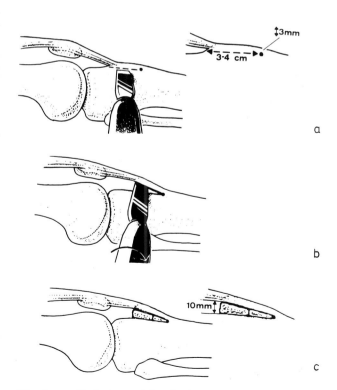

Fig. 5 a–c. Technique of the displacement forward

pierced in the frontal plane with the chisel 4–5 mm deep to its anterior margin and raised forward. Underneath, a corticocancellous block 1 cm in height from the iliac crest is inserted which is held fast when the tibial tuberosity springs back. For a more detailed description and information on follow-up treatment, see Bandi [2].

Results

Cases: To evaluate the results, we have a consecutive series of 100 patients who were operated on between 1966 and 1971. Fifty-six are men and 44 women; 86 patients underwent a personal clinical and radiological follow-up examination; 14 answered questionnaires.

Criteria for Evaluating the Results: The evaluation of the treatment results was based on a comparison of the preoperative and postoperative condition. An improvement to normal was marked 1 — with an increase by decimals depending on the existing residual complaints up to 2 which denoted no change. When the complaints were more severe than preoperatively, the mark increased to 3. The following criteria were marked according to this system:

1. Distance walking
2. Pain at rest
3. Pain while walking on level ground
4. Pain while ascending stairs
5. Pain while descending stairs
6. Uncertainty in walking (giving-way)
7. Recurrent effusions
8. Mobility
9. Fitness for work

From the sum of the nine marks, the arithmetic average was calculated. A result of 1–1.4 was marked good, 1.5–1.9 moderate, 2 unchanged, and results above 2 were marked poor.

We believe that we know the reason for the poor results. In two instances, we failed to correct a lateral displacement of the patella, in one case the indication for a knee operation was poor (simultaneous hip arthrosis). Two cases turned out to be PCP, and in the last case, the cause for the alleged severe pain was not found. If the same criteria are applied to the age group of 19–40 years, the following results were obtained:

No. of cases = 23, good = 20, moderate = 3
unchanged = 0 and poor = 0

Discussion

It is important that operative intervention not be left too late. We have attempted to determine a relationship between the objective findings (especially the characteristics of the arthrotic changes) and the symptoms during the observation period. The "increase" and "decrease" of the complaints provides information on the *course* of the disorder but not on its severity.

Table 6 lists changes in the subjective and objective results during the observation period. Groups 2 and 3 and 5 and 6 appear important to us with a total of 82% of the patients, whose pains either remained constant or improved, independent of the course of the arthrosis. They support our clinical experience that often patients with radiologically pronounced patellofemoral arthrosis have relatively few complaints, probably due to the relief from pressure caused by the displacement. For this reason, a patellectomy, as suggested by some authors in patellofemoral arthrosis, appears to be rarely indicated especially in the older age groups as they have great difficulty in regaining complete flexion. Based on the results presented, I consider it justifiable to continue to recommend an anterior displacement of the tibial tuberosity as the treatment of chondromalacia and patellofemoral arthrosis.

References

1. Aleman, O.: Chondromalacia of the patella. Acta chir. scand. **66,** 149 (1928)
2. Bandi, W.: Chondromalacia patellae und femoro-patellare Arthrose. Helv. chir. Acta, Suppl. **11,** 1972
3. Benninghoff, A.: Form und Bau der Gelenkknorpel in ihren Beziehungen zur Funktion. I. Mitteilung: Die modellierenden und formerhaltenden Faktoren des Knorpelreliefs. Z. Anat. Entwickl. Gesch. **76,** H. I./36 (1925)
4. Benninghoff, A.: 2. Teil: Der Aufbau des Knorpels in seinen Beziehungen zur Funktion. Z. Zellforsch. **2,** H. 5 (1925)
5. Benninghoff, A.: Der funktionelle Bau des Hyalinknorpels. Ergebn. Anat. Entwickl. Gesch. **26** (1925)
6. Blumensaat, C.: Die Lageabweichungen und Verrenkungen der Kniescheibe. Ergebn. Chir. **31,** 183 (1938)
7. Crooks, L. M.: Chondromalacia patellae. J. Bone Jt. Surg. **49 B,** 495 (1967)
8. Ficat, P.: Pathologie Femoro-patellaire. Paris: Masson 1970
9. Ficat, P.: Les Déséquilibres Rotuliens, de l'Hyperpression à l'Arthrose. Paris: Masson 1973
10. Fründ, H.: Traumatische Chondropathia der Patella, ein selbständiges Krankheitsbild. Zbl. Chir. **53,** 707 (1926)
11. Goymann, V., Müller, H. G.: New calculation of the biomechanics of the patellofemoral joint. Recent advances in basic research and clinical aspects. Proceedings of the internat. Congress, Rotterdam, Sept. 13–15, 1973, p. 16
12. Montmollin de, B.: Chondromalacie de la rotule. Rev. Orthop. **37,** 41 (1951)
13. Outerbridge, R. E.: The etiology of chondromalacia patellae. J. Bone Jt. Surg. **43 B,** 752 (1961)
14. Owre, A.: Chondromalacia patellae. Acta chir. scand. Suppl. **41,** 1 (1936)
15. Schneider, G.: Die Früharthrose im Femoropatellargelenk des Leistungssportlers. Ein Beitrag zur Pathogenese degenerativer Gelenkerkrankungen. Arch. orthop. Unfall-Chir. **54,** 401 (1968)
16. Viernstein, K., Weigert, M.: Chondromalacia patellae beim Leistungssportler. Z. Orthop. **104,** 432 (1969)
17. Zohlen, E.: Chondropathia patellae, über ihre Bedeutung u. Wesen. Bruns Beitr. klin. Chir. **69,** 174 (1942)

Translation from the German: Vorverlagerung der Tuberositas tibiae bei Chondromalacia patellae und femoro-patellarer Arthrose. In: Knorpelschaden am Knie, 4. Reisensburger Workshop zur klinischen Unfallchirurgie, edited by C. Burri and A. Rüter. In: Hefte zur Unfallheilkunde, Vol. 127 (1976). © Springer-Verlag 1976.

Subject Index

List of Contributors

Bandi, Prof. Dr. W.
Chirurgische Abteilung, Regionalspital, CH-3800 Interlaken, Switzerland

Baumann, Dr. D.
Orthopädische Klinik der Universität, Harlachinger Straße 51,
D-8000 München 90, Federal Republic of Germany

Burri, Prof. Dr. C.
Department für Chirurgie der Universität Ulm, Steinhövelstraße 9,
D-7900 Ulm, Federal Republic of Germany

Cotta, Prof. Dr. H.
Orthopädische Klinik der Universität, Schlierbacher Landstraße 200a,
D-6900 Heidelberg, Federal Republic of Germany

Ganz, Dr. R.
Orthopädische Universitätsklinik, CH-3010 Bern, Switzerland

Glinz, Dr. W.
Chirurgische Universitätsklinik B, CH-8006 Zürich, Switzerland

Gotzen, Dr. L.
Unfallchirurgische Klinik der Medizinischen Hochschule Karl-Wiechert-
Allee 9, D-3000 Hannover-Kleefeld, Federal Republic of Germany

Hackenbroch jun., Priv.-Doz. Dr. M. H.
Orthopädische Klinik der Universität, Harlachinger Straße 51,
D-8000 München 90, Federal Republic of Germany

Häring, Dr. M.
Abteilung für Unfallchirurgie der Chirurgischen Universitätsklinik,
Hugstetterstraße 55, D-7800 Freiburg, Federal Republic of Germany

Helbing, Dr. G.
Department für Chirurgie der Universität Ulm, Steinhövelstraße 9,
D-7900 Ulm, Federal Republic of Germany

Henche, Dr. H. R.
Kreiskrankenhaus Rheinfelden, Orthopädie-Abteilung,
D-7888 Rheinfelden/Baden, Federal Republic of Germany

Hertel, Dr. P.
Abteilung für Unfallchirurgie der Chirurgischen Universitätsklinik,
Ringstraße, D-6650 Homburg/Saar, Federal Republic of Germany

Hesse, Dr. I.
Unfallchirurgische Klinik der Medizinischen Hochschule, Karl-Wiechert-Allee 9, D-3000 Hannover-Kleefeld, Federal Republic of Germany

Hesse, Dr. W.
Unfallchirurgische Klinik der Medizinischen Hochschule, Karl-Wiechert-Allee 9, D-3000 Hannover-Kleefeld, Federal Republic of Germany

Kuner, Dr. E. H.
Abteilung für Unfallchirurgie der Chirurgischen Universitätsklinik, Hugstetterstraße 55, D-7800 Freiburg, Federal Republic of Germany

Leichs, Dr. L.
Orthopädische Klinik der Universität, Harlachinger Straße 51, D-8000 München 90, Federal Republic of Germany

Morscher, Prof. Dr. E.
Orthopädische Universitätsklinik, Basler Kinderspital, Römergasse 8, CH-4000 Basel, Switzerland

Müller, Priv.-Doz. Dr. J.
Chirurgische Klinik, Kantonsspital Liestal, Rheinstraße 26, CH-4410 Liestal, Switzerland

Müller, Dr. W.
Orthopädisch-Traumatologische Abteilung der Universitätskliniken, CH-4004 Basel, Switzerland

Muhr, Prof. Dr. G.
Unfallchirurgische Klinik der Medizinischen Hochschule, Karl-Wiechert-Allee 9, D-3000 Hannover-Kleefeld, Federal Republic of Germany

Puhl, Priv.-Doz. Dr. W.
Orthopädische Klinik der Universität, Schlierbacher Landstraße 200 a, D-6900 Heidelberg, Federal Republic of Germany

Refior, Priv.-Doz. Dr. H. J.
Orthopädische Klinik der Universität, Harlachinger Straße 51, D-8000 München 90, Federal Republic of Germany

Rehn, Prof. Dr. J.
Chirurgische Klinik der Berufsgenossenschaftlichen Krankenanstalten "Bergmannsheil", D-4630 Bochum, Federal Republic of Germany

Rüter, Priv.-Doz. Dr. A.
Department für Chirurgie der Universität Ulm, Steinhövelstraße 9, D-7900 Ulm, Federal Republic of Germany

Schneider, Dr. I.
Chirurgische Klinik der Berufsgenossenschaftlichen Krankenanstalten "Bergmannsheil", D-4630 Bochum, Federal Republic of Germany

Schweiberer, Prof. Dr. L.
Abteilung für Unfallchirurgie der Chirurgischen Universitätsklinik, Ringstraße,
D-6650 Homburg/Saar, Federal Republic of Germany

Spier, Prof. Dr. W., Wiss. Rat
Department für Chirurgie der Universität Ulm, Steinhövelstraße 9,
D-7900 Ulm, Federal Republic of Germany

Terbrüggen, Dr. D.
Abteilung für Unfallchirurgie der Universitätsklinik Freiburg,
Hugstetterstraße 55, D-7800 Freiburg, Federal Republic of Germany

Tscherne, Prof. Dr. H.
Unfallchirurgische Klinik der Medizinischen Hochschule, Karl-Wiechert-
Allee 9, D-3000 Hannover-Kleefeld, Federal Republic of Germany

Willenegger, Prof. Dr. H.
A.-O. Center, Murtenstraße 35, CH-3008 Bern, Switzerland

Springer AV Instruction Program

Slide Series

Internal Fixation – Basic Principles, Modern Means, Biomechanics

ASIF-Technique for Internal Fixation of Fractures

Internal Fixation of Patella and Malleolar Fractures

Total Hip Prostheses
Operation on Model and in vivo, Complications and Special Cases

Small Fragment Set Manual

Asepsis in Surgery

Films

Internal Fixation of Fractures:

Internal Fixation–Basic Principles and Modern Means

Internal Fixation of Forearm Fractures Internal Fixation of Noninfected

Diaphyseal Pseudarthroses

Internal Fixation of Malleolar Fractures

Internal Fixation of Patella Fractures

Medullary Nailing

Internal Fixation of the Distal End of the Humerus

Internal Fixation of Mandibular Fractures

Corrective Osteotomy of the Distal Tibia

The Biomechanics of Internal Fixation

Internal Fixation of Tibial Head Fractures
(in preparation)

Allo-Arthroplasty:

Total Hip Prostheses
(3 parts)
Part 1: Instruments. Operation on Model
Part 2: Operative Technique
Part 3: Complications. Special Cases

Elbow-Arthroplasty with the New GSB-Prosthesis

- ■ Further films and slide series in preparation
- ■ Technical data: 16 mm and super-8 (Eastmancolor, magnetic sound, optical sound), videocassettes. Slide series in ringbinders
- ■ All films in English or German, several in French; slide series with multilingual legends
- ■ Please ask for information material

Sales:
Springer-Verlag, Heidelberger Platz 3
D-1000 Berlin 33,
or
Springer-Verlag New York Inc.,
175 Fifth Avenue,
New York, NY 10010

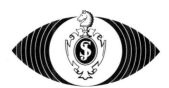

Springer-Verlag Berlin Heidelberg New York

Advances in Artificial Hip- and Knee-Joint Technology

Editors: M. Schaldach, D. Hohmann
In Collaboration with R. Thull, F. Hein
1976. 525 figures. XII, 525 pages
(Engineering in Medicine, Vol.2)
ISBN 3-540-07728-6

R. Bombelli

Osteoarthritis of the Hip

Pathogenesis and Consequent Therapy
With a Foreword by M.E. Müller
1976. 160 figures, 70 in color. X, 136 pages
ISBN 3-540-07842-8

P.G.J. Maquet

Biomechanics of the Knee

With Application to the Pathogenesis and the
Surgical Treatment of Osteoarthritis
1976. 184 figures. XIII, 230 pages
ISBN 3-540-07882-7

New Concepts in Maxillofacial Bone Surgery

Editor: B. Spiessl
With contributions by numerous experts.
1976. 183 figures, 36 tables. XIII, 194 pages
ISBN 3-540-07929-7

Progress in Orthopaedic Surgery

Editorial Board: N. Gschwend, D. Hohmann,
J.L. Hughes, D.S. Hungerford,
G.D. MacEwen, E. Morscher, J. Schatzker,
H. Wagner, U.H. Weil

Volume 1

Leg Length Discrepancy
The Injured Knee

Editor: D.S. Hungerford
With Contributions by numerous experts.
1977. 100 figures. X, 160 pages
ISBN 3-540-08037-6

Volume 2

Acetabular Dysplasia – Skeletal Dysplasias in Childhood

Edited by U.H. Weil
1977. 133 figures, 20 tables. IX, 200 pages
ISBN 3-540-08400-2

Journals

Anatomia clinica

(New in 1978 English & French edition)

Archives of Orthopaedic and Traumatic Surgery

(Continuation of "Archiv für orthopädische und Unfall-Chirurgie")

International Orthopaedics

Official Journal of the Societe Internationale de Chirurgie Orthopédique et de Traumatologie (SICOT)

World Journal of Surgery

Official Journal of the Societé Internationale de Chirurgie

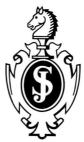

Springer-Verlag
Berlin
Heidelberg
New York